Take Back Control of Your Arthritis:
The 12 Critical Steps

Chlorzoxazon tab 500mg
sub for parafon fort
1 tab four (4) times daily

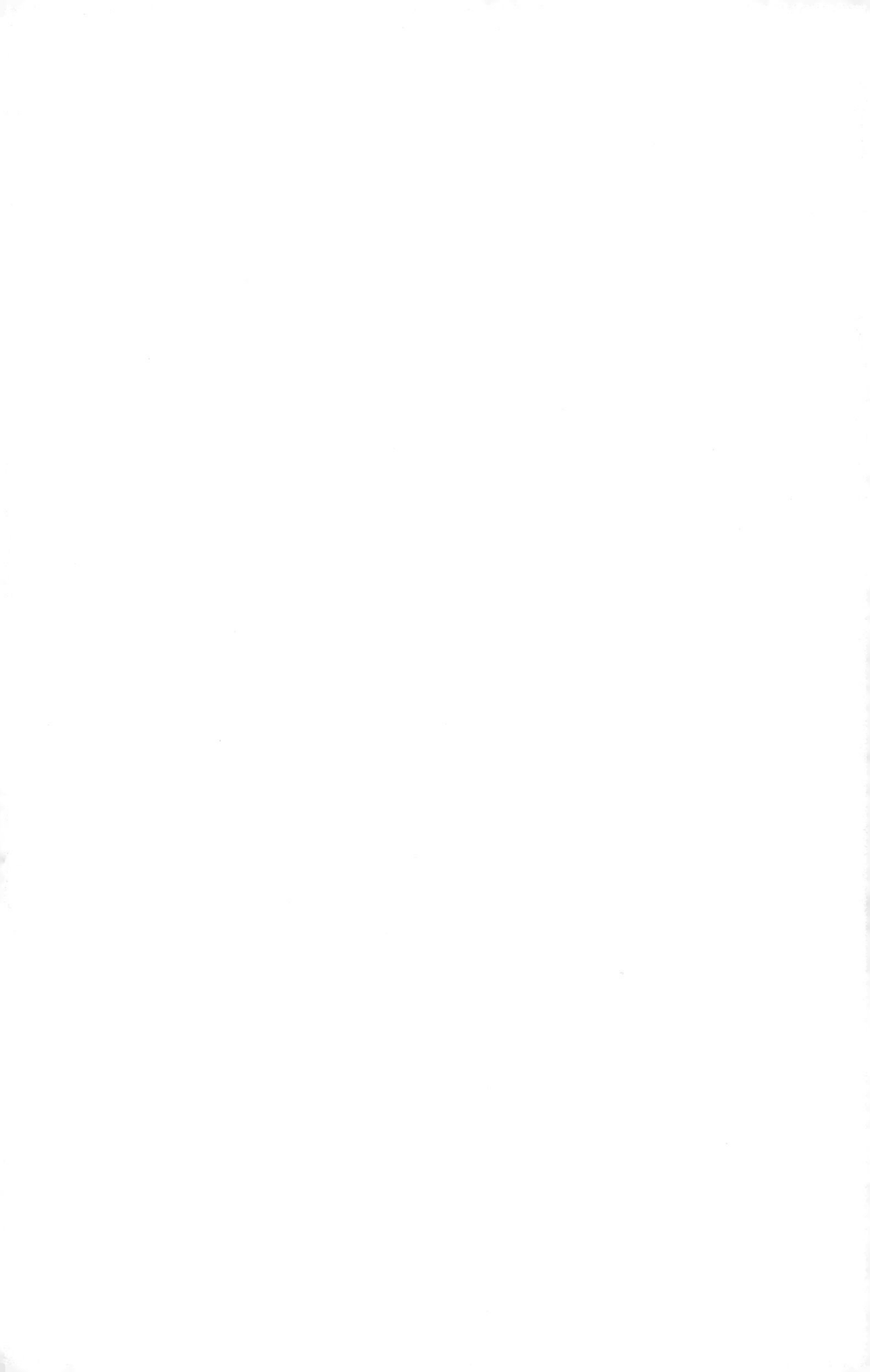

Take Back Control of Your Arthritis:

The 12 Critical Steps

Joel Rutstein M.D.

To order additional copies of this book, contact:
Xlibris Corporation
1-888-795-4274
www.Xlibris.com
Orders@Xlibris.com
23923

To my courageous and beautiful wife Barbara

Acknowledgements

I would like to thank Diana Garcia for her transcription help in preparing the manuscript for this book. I also appreciate the editing assistance from Sima and Lyle Wolf, Judy Gerstein, Larry and Ronna Rutstein, and Dr. Rodolfo Molina. The book would never have been published without the special efforts of Jason and Randi Marks.

Important Disclaimer

This book is written to enlighten and inspire you. Any recommendations by the author should first be discussed with your own physician before implementing them. Since many of these therapies have the potential for causing complications or side effects, you should be monitored by your personal physician when undertaking any of these treatments for your condition.

The author wishes to disclose that he has served as a consultant and clinical researcher for many pharmaceutical and health-related companies over the years. He has received financial compensation for his time and effort involved in these activities. These companies include Amgen, BioniCare, Johnson and Johnson, Merck, Pfizer, Pharmacia, Purdue Frederick, and Wyeth Pharmaceuticals. The author does not have any stock ownership or other financial interest in any of these companies.

The author's opinions and recommendations, however, are his own and are the result of over twenty-five years of clinical practice in the field of rheumatology. This experience has been combined with his knowledge and appreciation of the available scientific information and medical literature that support these ideas.

About the Author

Dr. Joel Rutstein is the creator and producer of ArthritisCentral.com, one of the most comprehensive websites dealing with arthritis and osteoporosis and designed for patient self-education. He is a board-certified rheumatologist and Director of the Arthritis Diagnostic and Treatment Center in San Antonio, Texas, where he has been in clinical practice for over twenty-five years. His clinic is one of the largest full-service arthritis centers in the United States. Dr. Rutstein also serves as Clinical Professor of Medicine at the University of Texas Health Science Center (UTHSC). Following the completion of both his undergraduate and medical training at the University of Pennsylvania in Philadelphia, Dr. Rutstein relocated to San Antonio after being drafted into the U.S. Army to teach at the Academy of Health Sciences at Ft. Sam Houston. Following a two-year fellowship in rheumatology at the UTHSC, Dr. Rutstein began his clinical practice in 1978. He is past president of the Texas Rheumatism Association and has been honored with the Humanitarian of the Year Award by the South Texas Arthritis Foundation. Dr. Rutstein has also helped produce multiple full-length patient educational video programs, which are available at ArthritisMall.com.

Contents

STEP 7: TAKE BACK CONTROL OF YOUR LIFESTYLE 153

STEP 8: TAKE BACK CONTROL OF YOUR WORK SITUATION 177

Introduction

Within days of a spectacular Fourth of July fireworks display that my wife and I watched while embracing one another, our lives were suddenly shattered. My wife had gone in for a CAT scan to clarify some lower abdominal discomfort that she had been experiencing. This turned out to be much ado about nothing, but an incidental finding was the presence of a nodule astutely noted in the lower lung. Following a needle biopsy, she and I were totally devastated when the pathologist informed us that my wife had lung cancer. She subsequently underwent surgery to remove the lower lobe of her lung, and this was then followed by chemotherapy and radiation treatments. As I write this introductory chapter, my wife and I still have no idea of whether the treatment will work or not. Our lives have been turned upside down. All of our trips and other plans have been cancelled. We live one day at a time, not knowing when my wife will wake up and have a "good" day or when she will feel miserable with marked fatigue, trouble swallowing, nausea, or other consequences of her treatments. I find myself fighting intermittent feelings of extreme anxiety and even some depression in trying to deal with what is happening and yet wanting to be very supportive of what she is going through.

I am sure that many of you can relate to this story. For some of you, it was being told that you had a significant form of arthritis that changed your life. Once extremely active, you now may be more limited in your activities and forced to deal with the side effects of numerous potent medications. For still others, it may have been a diagnosis of systemic lupus erythematosus that has cast a shadow over your previously happy outlook. Now you have to cope with the uncertainty of when you might experience a flare-up of this condition. You worry about potential involvement of your kidneys or central nervous system. If you were an "outdoors" type of person, now you are limited as to your sun exposure and need to use a strong sun block if and when you do briefly go outside. Others may have had to learn to cope with the chronic and diffuse pain associated with fibromyalgia syndrome. Your tolerance for physical activity may now be markedly restricted by your degree of muscle pain or fatigue. Perhaps you are a patient with osteoarthritis, who has recently been told that you are "bone on bone" in your hips or knees and that you will need joint replacement surgery if you are to walk without pain in the future. Without the surgery, you are faced with the possibility of being incapacitated and totally dependent on others to get by. I could go on and on with other similar predicaments that people with rheumatic diseases are facing on a daily basis all over the world.

Pain is certainly the most significant common denominator in these rheumatic disorders. When I was a medical school student at the University of Pennsylvania in Philadelphia, I awoke one morning with the worst pain that I had ever experienced. It was over my right flank radiating down into my right groin. The pain was so severe that I was nearly run over trying to flag down a car on Spruce Street to get someone to drive me to the hospital. It turned out that I was trying to pass a kidney stone, which I succeeded in doing after being administered intravenous narcotics in the emergency room. Since then, I have had other similar recurrent episodes characterized by acute and excruciating pain requiring emergency room treatment before subsiding. Some people say that the pain of childbirth is the worst pain that a person can experience. Obviously I have no personal means of comparison just having been an interested bystander when my wife gave birth to my lovely daughters. I must admit that it certainly looked painful enough to me, but kidney stones have got to be a close second as far as the degree of pain involved. On a scale of zero to ten on a pain scale, I would have to put it at a twelve! Over the years, I learned first-hand what it is like to try to convince a reluctant doctor of the severity of pain I was feeling and the need for stronger doses of potent medicine to relieve my agony. Physicians, who have never even been ill, and certainly those who have never had to deal with intense pain, tend to act like a bunch of "doubting Thomases." They often are judgmental and may only begrudgingly give small and inadequate doses of pain medicine that still leave you hurting.

Does this sound familiar to you? How many times have you encountered a doctor who doesn't seem to take your pain seriously and gives you prescriptions that hardly put a dent in your level of pain? Prior studies have borne this out showing that physicians, as a group, often under-treat pain. New hospital guidelines now require that patients be assessed regularly with evaluation of the level or degree of severity of their pain. This information may help to compel doctors to do a better job of treating pain.

Now, you may be wondering why I have spent so much time telling you about my own personal situation and even a part of my medical history. The reason is that I want you to understand from the "get-go" that I can totally relate to what you are going through in your life. I am aware of how illness can affect your life, how it can destroy relationships and families, how it can ruin your career, and how it can throw you into a "depressed state." I empathize with the pain you are feeling and would be thrilled to be able to convey helpful information to lessen it for you.

In addition to my personal first-hand experiences in dealing with pain and the stress and consequences of coping with illness in my own family, I also am able to draw on the knowledge gained by over twenty-five years of patient care in the field of rheumatology. During that time span, I founded and have served as director of the Arthritis Diagnostic and Treatment Center in San Antonio, Texas. The center, one of the largest in the United States, now has seven full time rheumatologists catering to all the different forms of rheumatic disease. As Clinical Professor of Medicine at the University of Texas Health Science Center in San Antonio, I am called upon to teach medical students about the practice of rheumatology and to hone their skills in the physical examination of patients with rheumatic conditions. This encourages me to clarify my own thinking about rheumatic diseases. It helps me improve my ability to explain different concepts and principles in educating patients as well. My participation in ongoing clinical research studies involving revolutionary treatments enables me to remain at the forefront of all of the exciting breakthroughs that are occurring in the field of rheumatology. No "book-knowledge" or research, however, can ever serve as a substitute for the hands-on experience of caring for thousands of individuals with arthritis and osteoporosis. I have learned so much by carefully listening to my patients' symptoms and their response or lack of response to various remedies. I have also gained tremendous insight into their personal lives and the impact that their rheumatic conditions have had on every aspect of their existence. This book, therefore, is a compilation of all that I have gleaned not only from my studies over the years, but also from my actual patient encounters and experiences.

Arthritis can be a devastating illness. It can cause severe and incapacitating pain. Over a period of years it can lead to deformity and eventual disability. This may result in an inability to hold down a job and earn a living. Financial pressures may put an enormous strain on a marriage and lead to an unhappy home environment or possibly divorce. Some forms of arthritis may even be associated with significant internal organ involvement, which could be disastrous if not managed correctly. So even though cancer and heart disease often get bigger headlines in the press, arthritis can be just as debilitating if you are the one afflicted with it. It is also a more common health problem than many people appreciate. It is estimated that seventy million people in the U.S. alone have a form of arthritis. Another twenty to thirty million individuals are affected by osteoporosis. When the direct medical costs of care are combined with the indirect costs of lost wages due to disability, arthritis ranks near the top of the list of financial drains on our health resources.

Take Back Control of Your Arthritis: The 12 Critical Steps provides the arthritis patient with the essential measures that a person needs to take control of their rheumatic disease. This book provides you with a clear directional road map of what is required in order to try to conquer your illness. Since there are over one hundred different forms of rheumatic disease, not every single step may apply to every specific condition. There are, however, enough areas in common to make this step-wise approach to controlling a person's arthritic condition useful to everyone affected.

You may wonder when I speak of taking back control of your arthritis, from what or whom are you regaining control? In most cases, you are really just finding highly effective ways of counteracting the natural progression of the disease. If left unopposed, an inflammatory arthritic disorder could lead to destruction and erosion of bones at the joint, as well as contributing to joint space narrowing. Many patients, however, are unaware of the exciting changes in treatment that have occurred in just the last five years that can dramatically alter the outcome of even the most aggressive forms of inflammatory arthritis. One of the 12 critical steps presented in this book will deal with biologic agents that are revolutionizing the treatment of arthritis as we enter the new millennium. In taking back control, arthritis sufferers can begin asserting themselves to a greater degree in their own treatment programs and assume a greater responsibility for their own destiny.

Of the 12 critical steps, the first two deal with doctor related issues. In Step 1, I will start off by spending some time discussing the process of finding the right physician for you. You will not be able to conquer your arthritis without the help and support of a knowledgeable doctor. Thus, it becomes essential that the doctor who is treating your rheumatic disease is the best one for you. If you have a very mild form of arthritis, you may do well with treatment by your primary care physician. If you have more significant arthritis or a more complex rheumatic illness, then I will explain to you in Step 2 why it so critically important that you place yourself in the hands of the best rheumatologist available in your geographic location. Since there are only several thousand rheumatologists in the entire country, it is not possible for all seventy million patients with arthritis to be seen by a rheumatologist. I will still make the case, however, as to why patients treated by a rheumatologist tend to have better outcomes. Then I will leave it up to you as to whether you feel that you would be better off being treated by a rheumatology specialist or not.

In Steps 3 and 4, I will explore issues related to controlling pain and inflammation. Pain is often not adequately addressed or sufficiently treated by physicians. I will describe many of the treatment options currently available to you. The subject of how to better control the inflammation caused by arthritis will also include information on the new COX-2 inhibitors (Celebrex, Vioxx, and Bextra) as well as over-the-counter medicines. If you are to regain a greater sense of control over your disease, then you also need to be aware of important issues regarding the safety of these medications.

Step 5 will address the whole new area of treatment with biologic therapy, which probably is the most exciting development in the field of rheumatology in the last fifty years. I will bring you up-to-date on the tumor necrosis factor inhibitors, Remicade, Enbrel, and Humira. I will also familiarize you with the Interleukin-1 (IL-1) inhibitor Kineret. Disease-modifying treatments may serve an important role as the backbone of therapy to which a biologic treatment is added. This is particularly true of the use of methotrexate in the treatment of rheumatoid arthritis and psoriatic arthritis. Various disease-modifying anti-rheumatic drugs (DMARDs), including methotrexate, will be discussed as part of Step 5.

Step 6 will deal with the issue of medication and treatment costs. I will also discuss my opinions on the expense and value of over-the-counter remedies. It would be shortsighted of me in helping you to regain control over your arthritis (with its ramifications on your home and work life) not to consider cost issues.

This leads us to Step 7, which deals with the important subject of lifestyle modification. Many of you, I suspect, would prefer to have just one critical step to conquer to take back control of your arthritis. Wouldn't it be great if that step just required that your doctor prescribed a "magic pill" and your arthritis completely and miraculously disappeared forever! Unfortunately this is not available yet, even though in some cases the new biologic response modifiers have had a fairly dramatic impact on the natural course of arthritis. It would certainly be easier to take a panacea, rather then to be forced to make important lifestyle changes that you may find odious. The issues of smoking, coffee, and alcohol consumption will all be addressed. If you are to take control of your rheumatic condition, then you will need to be more knowledgeable about how to balance your activity level with the right amount of rest. Your spiritual side also needs to be discussed, and concepts regarding spiritual self-healing will be touched upon. Many arthritis patients who are in the early stages of their disease are still in denial. They have not yet come to grips with what will be required of them in order to help arrest their condition.

In the workplace, many arthritis sufferers are reluctant to complain about their workload or a lack of accommodation to their particular needs. This may be partly due to fears about being terminated from the job if their supervisor becomes more aware of their condition. The patient may worry that his or her boss may misinterpret requests for work modification as implying a poor work attitude or an inability to perform the work in an acceptable manner. For those of you still working, it will not be possible for you to truly take back control of your arthritis without dealing with such issues as an ergonomically correct work setting, reasonable work hours, activity levels on the job, and stress associated with work. These will all be discussed as part of Step 8.

Step 9 deals with taking back control of your exercise program with strengthening and conditioning to help counteract the effects of your arthritis on your muscles and joints. There are a great many misconceptions about what constitutes healthy and beneficial exercise. You may have received various exercise recommendations from lay individuals, who may mean well but who may actually be pushing you into doing things that may be incorrect. Patients often don't understand the difference between abusive activities and therapeutic exercise. Therefore, in Step 9 I will try to map out some important points to enable you to personally take back control of your exercise with the right program for you.

Many patients may experience anxiety and/or depression in connection with a rheumatic condition. Step 10 will deal with taking back control of your emotions. Practically all patients with significant rheumatic disease, no matter what their socio-economic background or level of education, will experience transient or more persistent depression at some time during the course of their illness. Nighttime pain or uncontrolled feelings of anxiety may lead to interrupted sleep. A lack of restful sleep may then contribute to changes in mood. It is extremely important to discuss ways for you to regain control of your emotional state in order to increase the likelihood of feeling better. This will then provide you with the proper mental outlook to accomplish many of the other steps in this twelve-step program.

One of the very best ways to feel well and less depressed is to have satisfying sex. Sexual orgasms release natural substances in the brain called endorphins, which can diminish pain sensations. Having someone who can caress you softly and tenderly boosts your self-esteem and decreases your feelings of being isolated from the rest of the world by your physical limitations and inadequacies. Step 11, therefore, addresses the importance of taking back control of your sex life. In this chapter, I include topics such as helpful tips about sexual positions and the use of sexual aids. I also address practical issues such as the timing of your sexual activity and important considerations about the effects of medications on your ability to enjoy sex.

This book is part of a larger plan to inform rheumatic disease patients about how to better cope with their medical conditions. I have also created one of the largest patient information web sites on arthritis and osteoporosis at ArthritisCentral.com. It houses numerous videos dealing with arthritis and osteoporosis. I have previously written another book entitled *Combatting Pain and Arthritis with Answers That Could Change Your Life*, which answers patients' specific questions about the most common forms of rheumatic diseases. I certainly place a high priority on patient education as one of the most important weapons patients can utilize to fight back against their rheumatic disorder. Step 12, therefore, is devoted to taking back control of your self-education and enlightening you on how to gain access to up-to-date helpful medical information. Knowledge empowers you to do many things that can maximize your treatment outcome. Knowledge also helps you to avoid the pitfalls that may impede your path towards achieving better control of your condition. Hopefully all of the knowledge that you gain from this book and from becoming familiar with the 12 critical steps involved in taking back control of your arthritis will enable you to improve your life and decrease your pain and suffering. If that happens, it would be wonderful for you and most gratifying to me.

Step 1: Find a Doctor You Can Trust

Telltale Signs That You Are Having Problems with Your Personal or Primary Care Physician:

- Your doctor always seems so distant from you.

- Your doctor is rude to you.

- Your doctor gets angry with you if you don't follow every one of his/her recommendations precisely.

- Your doctor gets upset with you if you question him/her about the rationale for the physician's specific treatment recommendation.

- Your doctor doesn't listen to you.

- Your doctor doesn't address all of your symptoms.

- Your doctor doesn't seem interested in you as a person.

- Your doctor is never available for emergencies.

- Your doctor keeps you waiting forever, and then rushes through your visit.

- Your doctor doesn't explain things to you in a clear, easily understandable way.

- Your doctor tells you that it's all in your head.

Searching

In our teenage years, we already are thinking about the

qualities we would like to find in the perfect spouse, lover, or significant other. Falling in love is often a wonderful "accident" with romantic feelings that can't always be clearly delineated. Yet, for most of us there is definitely a list of characteristics we would love to find in the right individual. Making a lifelong commitment is a huge step and taking one's time to make the right choice is extremely important. This is the person with whom you will share the most private thoughts and feelings, as well as your greatest joys. This person will help you raise a family and support you in your efforts to be successful and find happiness in your life. So the search for the right person is one of the most critical endeavors you will ever undertake.

This effort to find the right partner contrasts sharply with the time and energy ordinarily devoted to finding your personal physician. This is the person you entrust with decisions that could determine whether you live or die. You may discuss things with your doctor that you do not even want to disclose to your spouse, especially when it comes to bowel or bladder functions, or problems with sexual performance. Yet I see a large number of patients in my practice who are enrolled in managed care plans where their primary care physician is simply assigned to them. Other patients often will select their primary doctor based on how close to their home he or she is located. Obviously convenience is an important consideration, but it should not take precedence over other much more important factors, which I will describe below. You would think that the selection of such an important person in your life would deserve as least as much time and energy as you put in when considering which motor vehicle or home you wish to purchase.

Since most rheumatic conditions are long-term problems, the relationship with your personal physician over many years may end up being similar to a marriage. As with a spouse or significant other, there is probably a "perfect" physician match somewhere out there waiting for you. Your first encounter with your doctor should be evaluated much like your assessment after a first date. If he/she is not pleasant then, it should act as a clue to you that things might not get much better down the road. Occasionally you may get more comfortable with some doctors over time, but first impressions should not necessarily be ignored. As in a marriage, if the relationship with your primary care physician is not going well, then you may need to get "divorced," and go out and find a better match for you. If you are unhappy with the way you are being treated, don't drag it out. You need to change to a physician who inspires confidence and trust, someone who acts in a professional manner and is caring towards you.

The Ideal Physician for You

If you are going to take back control of your arthritis, then you must start by having the ideal personal physician available who is best suited for your personality and your medical condition. This individual may have a great deal of influence over your destiny and medical treatment. In an HMO, for example, a primary care doctor may be in control of whether you get referred to a rheumatologist who specializes in the rheumatic diseases. Your primary care physician may also decide if he/she will consent to your having various studies or physical therapy treatments. If you wind up with a doctor who is in an adversarial relationship with you and is essentially working against your best interests, then you will wind up being victimized in the process.

When I first went into medical practice, I was told about the "three A's." The "three A's" stand for the words "able," "affable," and "available." When a doctor first gets out of residency and fellowship and is preparing for clinical practice, he/she tends to think that "able" is the most important of these three "A's" in determining future success. Surprisingly, it is whether you are "affable" or likeable that turns out to be the most important of the three. Next in importance is whether you are "available" or accessible. It is not very helpful to patients if the physician is extremely bright, but is booked for months and, therefore, cannot evaluate a new patient or an established patient with an emergency. Interestingly, being "able" or knowledgeable is third in importance. Patients have a great deal of difficulty being able to judge a physician's true level of knowledge or skill, but it is quite obvious to them whether the doctor is pleasant and caring. In a physician's training the emphasis is definitely on becoming "able" with an enormous amount of factual information and skills taught to each medical student, intern, and resident. Not much time is devoted to learning how to be a more caring healer and more compassionate doctor.

Sometimes a lack of "availability" can be misleading, however, since a very special and personable physician may be extraordinarily busy due to his/her wonderful reputation. This type of doctor is unlikely to have many patients switching to another physician due to dissatisfaction. A high percentage of established patients in this practice, therefore, will be retained and will keep the schedule filled. It should alarm you if you go to a doctor, who has been in practice for a number of years, and you find the waiting room empty and his/her schedule wide open. This is often a sign that patients are not coming back for follow-up visits once they have had one or more disappointing encounters with this physician. It's the same principle as finding a restaurant completely empty on a Saturday night. How good could the food and service be? You should ask yourself the same question if the doctor you are seeing is not at all busy (unless he or she is just starting out in practice).

Being likeable or affable also can sometimes be deceiving. There are some doctors who are "charmers." Some physicians can "con" you with their sweetness and kindness, but it turns out that it is all a façade. This is why it is imperative to get other opinions from other physicians and patients under this doctor's care, to validate your choice of doctors. Arthritis support groups, exercise and aquatics classes, and church and synagogue gatherings are some examples of good places to accumulate reliable information from other people about the top physicians in your community.

Qualities to Look for in a Doctor

I think that it is important for me to give you a behind-the-scenes discussion and perspective about physicians that is rarely conveyed to patients. How else can I help you to select the right physician for your needs? So much of what follows in Steps 2 through 12 depends in large measure on Step 1—finding a doctor whom you can trust. Therefore, I need to explore all of the characteristics of a quality physician so that you have some better parameters to follow in making your choice.

Whenever a doctor sees you, whether in the office or hospital, a medical history will be elicited from you. It is important that your physician is a good listener and allows you to adequately tell your story. You may be able to tell whether or not the doctor is listening intently by his/her facial expressions, or by some nodding of the head in agreement. If your MD does not appear to be focused or interested in what you are recounting, this is a bad sign. It is appropriate for your doctor to be recording notes about your history, so the fact that he/she is writing while you are speaking is acceptable. Your physician should still be making eye contact with you in between the note taking. A poor listener will interrupt you frequently, sometimes even causing you to lose your train of thought. You may even feel hurried or pressed by rapid-fire questions as you attempt to describe your symptoms in your own way. If a physician asks you something that you have already covered, then he/she may not be concentrating on what you are saying.

Once your history has been obtained, the next step is the

performance of a physical examination. It is important to find a doctor who is gentle, rather than rough. Patients with arthritis are hurting, and an examination of your joints can be quite painful if it is done in a highly aggressive way. It is a good sign if your doctor apologizes to you if he/she causes you some discomfort during the course of this examination. This is a clear demonstration of his or her concern about the pain you are feeling. Be wary of a physician who "forces" your joints beyond a comfortable range of motion, thus inducing an increased amount of pain. It is, therefore, best if your physician has "soft" hands and examines you in a way that demonstrates a genuine concern for the painful condition you have delineated in your history.

There are other helpful hints about this physician that may come out during a physical. Is the doctor concerned about your comfort level as you sit in a skimpy gown in a freezing cold room? The physician may summon a nurse to turn the heat up, or request a blanket to warm you up. Does the doctor show care in keeping the private parts of your body adequately covered, except when being examined? Does the physician put out a helping hand to assist you down from the exam table, or are you left to fend for yourself while the doctor retreats to his/her desk? When a doctor gives you some support as you step down from an examining table, it shows a real concern about your well being in making sure that you do not fall and injure yourself. It is a subtle message that the doctor genuinely cares.

Once the history and physical examination have been completed, it is time for the physician to begin to explain what he /she thinks is causing your problems, what tests might need to be run, and what remedies are available to help you. This is your opportunity to assess the communication skills of this physician. Are things being explained to you in a clear and understandable way? Make sure that the doctor is not using complicated and incomprehensible medical jargon that is designed to impress you, but goes completely above your head. Also, is the doctor taking the time to explain things at a slow enough pace so that you can absorb all of the information that is being given to you? You need to realize that your anxiety about what might be happening to your body due to your medical problems may interfere with your ability to listen and comprehend everything the doctor is saying.

It is extremely undesirable to have a primary care physician who does not take the time to explain things carefully to you. A doctor who has problems communicating may be curt or short with you. Some doctors may simply hand you a prescription for a medication without ever really explaining why you need to take it or what they thought was wrong with you. Also, whenever you are prescribed a new medicine, a good communicator will discuss the benefits and potential side effects so that you will know what to expect when taking it.

It is best to find a doctor who has a positive and upbeat outlook towards you and your condition. This is an individual who tries to put a hopeful and positive "spin" on your chances for improvement. He/she may point out examples of other patients in his/her own practice or in the medical literature who have done well with a particular form of treatment. This can be very encouraging to a worried patient. A doctor who always seems to dwell on the negative or "downside" of things can become quite depressing for the patient. It is certainly hard enough to maintain one's optimism in the face of some chronic disease, and more so if your doctor is constantly painting a bleak picture for you. This is not to say that your doctor should not be honest with you, but there are ways to do this without destroying any feelings of hope that you still harbor.

Some doctors' personalities are not always a good "fit" for patients with chronic rheumatic diseases. The natural course of many forms of arthritis and musculo-skeletal disease is to wax and wane. Patients may be on a proverbial roller coaster, at times suffering severe worsening of their health status, and then weeks or months later feeling markedly improved. Some physicians may become quite frustrated with the chronic and recurrent nature of these problems. The fact that they cannot totally and permanently control the patient's symptoms may become aggravating and may be a blow to their ego. This may then be expressed to the patient in the form of anger or irritation—as if the patient were in some way responsible for the fact that he/she had not shown greater improvement. It is far better to find a physician who looks forward to the challenges of chronic diseases, and is not so readily frustrated by the patient's relapses.

Ideally, you want to find a physician who is kind. This is a doctor who will comfort you when you are suffering, someone who will sit at your bedside and hold your hand to give you strength and support. This physician will provide you with plenty of "TLC"—tender, loving care. There are many doctors out there who have adequate medical knowledge in their particular field, but they lack the compassion that patients crave and need. Contrary to most patients' expectations, some doctors may come across as "hard" or unfeeling. Rarely, a patient will encounter a physician who is actually mean. If the patient does not adhere to every medical recommendation exactly, then this particular type of doctor is infuriated and may verbally reprimand the patient.

Unfortunately, some physicians see themselves as almost "God-like" in importance, and any challenge to their knowledge and authority becomes a personal threat to them. If you question their judgment or recommendations, they may respond or subsequently treat you in a cold and calloused manner. This contrasts with a physician who sees himself as more of a humanitarian, available to render care and advise you intelligently, but still respectful of your right to participate in decisions about your health care. In the hands of this type of doctor, you feel as if you are being treated like a family member.

It is best if you can find an MD who is open-minded to new or alternative (complementary) treatments. The pain and frustration that arthritis sufferers experience can often drive patients to experiment with novel or unproven remedies. A good doctor will try to steer you through this "minefield" so you avoid hurting yourself by taking something that might be dangerous to your health. What you don't need is someone getting angry with you for considering some other mode of treatment out of a sense of desperation. A physician who is close-minded will not be willing to consider ancillary alternative treatments that may complement traditional forms of therapy. You need to find a doctor who is knowledgeable enough to correctly advise you, but at the same time compassionate enough to understand why you are constantly searching for some new way to better control your painful symptoms.

Knowledge and skill are still very important attributes of a great doctor, and I do not mean to minimize them. Your doctor should preferably have been trained in a top medical institution and be board-certified in his/her area of expertise. It is, however, extremely difficult for you, the patient, to be able to accurately assess the degree of knowledge that your doctor possesses. Other physicians in the medical community will most likely be aware of your doctor's abilities, but this information would be hard for you to obtain unless you have some physician-friends. You may be able to find out from the office staff if the doctor has published articles in his specialty. It would be encouraging to know that your doctor goes away periodically to attend national medical meetings and seminars to receive the latest updates on changes in medical therapy. If you bring articles from health magazines or the Internet into your doctor visits for clarification and discussion, you may also be able to tell from the physician's response if he is knowledgeable about the latest developments concerning your medical condition.

You would like to have a doctor who demonstrates a strong

work ethic and is devoted to his medical practice. It is, of course, healthy for your physician to take personal time off periodically in order to feel renewed and be able to cope with the huge responsibilities of running a medical practice. Yet, you would not want to get the feeling that your doctor was intrinsically lazy, or always complaining about how overloaded and overwhelmed he/she was with the workload. Also, it would not be very comforting to know that every time you seemed to be in need of your doctor, he/she was off gallivanting about on some far off trip and never there for you. At a minimum, if your doctor were taking a well-deserved vacation, you would want to be reassured that another quality physician was available for you in the event of an emergency.

One important but sometimes-neglected way of coping with pain is with humor. Finding a doctor who has a good sense of humor is an added bonus. He/she may be able to help you keep things in better perspective and not fall into a feeling of total despair. Using humor to counteract pain and depression can be uplifting and even therapeutic. In the writings of Norman Cousins in the *Saturday Evening Post*, we learned about his frustrations with a form of arthritis called ankylosing spondylitis, and how he "laughed" himself back to health using humor.

In the end, the most important thing in selecting your personal physician is finding someone who really cares. You want to be putting your health in the hands of someone who is concerned about your pain and suffering, who values your input and opinions, and who totally empathizes with the havoc your medical condition is causing in your life. If you can find such a person who is extremely knowledgeable as well, then you have indeed lucked out and you should stay "married" to that physician as long as possible.

Nowadays it is getting more difficult to find all of these traits in doctors because of the "burn-out" that currently plagues the medical profession. The advent of managed care along with government intrusions into medical practices have placed enormous additional burdens and added frustration onto doctors' lives. Some physicians have actually quit practicing, rather than deal with the loss of control of the decision-making process in caring for patients. Others have had to work much longer hours to make do because of cutbacks in some reimbursement while facing continually increasing overhead expenses. The paperwork requirements for documenting patient encounters have expanded significantly. All of these time drains only serve to take away from the additional time that the doctor could be spending with the patient, rather than with administrative type duties. This results in a doctor feeling squeezed by the system, a doctor who now feels robbed of the joy of practicing medicine and the art of healing that he or she once cherished. So finding a personal physician who has been able to withstand all of these outside forces in medicine can be even more of a challenge these days.

Although it may involve some effort to find the right personal physician for you, it will be well worth it. You must have a great doctor as your ally if you plan to take back control of your arthritis. All of the steps that follow in the ensuing chapters will require the knowledge and support of a caring physician, partnering with you in your effort to deal with your condition. It is imperative that you establish a relationship with a physician whom you can totally trust and count upon no matter what the situation. Finding the perfect personal physician for you is, therefore, the first and essential cornerstone of your twelve-step plan to take back control of your arthritis.

Key Points in Finding a Physician You Can Trust:

1. Make sure to put some time and effort into finding the right primary doctor for you and your medical condition.

2. First impressions of a doctor are often valid and should not be ignored, if negative.

3. If the relationship is not right, then be willing to sever it and move on.

4. It is best if your doctor is affable, but don't be deceived by "charmers."

5. Try to find a doctor who is a good listener.

6. Find a doctor who is gentle, kind, and compassionate.

7. Find a physician who communicates to you in a clear and understandable manner and is not trying to impress you with big words and fancy scientific language.

8. Find a doctor who conveys a positive outlook and gives you a hopeful, optimistic feeling. A sense of humor about life can also be helpful in coping.

9. Find a physician who is open-minded about new or alternative (complementary) forms of treatment and does not seem threatened by your questions or personal research relating to your condition.

10. Consider yourself most fortunate if you can find a doctor who combines many of these elements with a vast amount of knowledge and skill.

Step 2: Find a Rheumatologist

Telltale Signs That You Need to Find a Rheumatologist:

- Your primary care physician seems confused by your illness.

- Your primary care physician rarely injects your joints with medication when you have a flare-up of your arthritis.

- Your primary care physician tells you that he or she can handle all of your medical problems, including your arthritis, just as well as any specialist.

- Your primary care physician has never mentioned or ever recommended physical therapy or a specific exercise program.

- You have active inflammatory arthritis, such as rheumatoid arthritis, but you have only been treated with typical anti-inflammatory medications for years.

- You have active arthritis but have never had x-rays of your involved joints.

- Every time that you complain of any aches or pains, your regular physician responds by ordering more lab tests.

- Your regular doctor implies that much of your problem is imagined or "in your mind."

- Your personal physician suggests that a large part of your pain is due to the fact that you are depressed.

- Your primary care physician implies that he or she feels that you are not in that much pain and that you are overusing your pain medication. You feel, however, that your pain is not well controlled.

What's a Rheumatologist and Why Bother?

Over the years, life's experiences teach us how to respond in the event of an emergency. If the toilet gets completely stopped up, then we call a plumber before we end up flooding our bathroom floor. If the brakes in the car aren't functioning correctly, then we drive the vehicle carefully to the local mechanic before we end up in an accident that is easily avoidable.

In the medical field, most people know that if they are experiencing chest pain with possible heart problems that they should be seen by a cardiologist before they go on to have a full-blown heart attack. If a person falls and fractures a hip, he would want an orthopedic surgeon called in to operate and not a urologist or ENT specialist. Yet when it comes to arthritis, many individuals are still unaware that there is a specialist available to treat these conditions called a rheumatologist. Like the plumber and auto mechanic in the above examples, the rheumatologist has the knowledge and skills to keep you out of trouble before your arthritis progresses and causes you significant disability. If you intend to take back control of your arthritis, then you are going to have to find the best rheumatologist in your area and start consulting with that physician as soon as possible.

Why a rheumatologist, you may ask? A rheumatologist is a medical doctor who specializes in musculo-skeletal illnesses including all forms of arthritis, connective tissue diseases, autoimmune conditions, spinal disorders, and osteoporosis. A rheumatologist does not normally perform surgery in an operating room (except for the rare rheumatologist who is doing arthroscopic surgery of the knee). The training involved to become a rheumatology specialist includes completion of a medical internship followed by a two-year residency specializing in internal medicine (adult medical conditions). The individual then takes a certification exam to become board-certified in internal medicine under the auspices of the American College of Physicians. The doctor then has to complete a two-year fellowship in rheumatology followed by yet another certification exam. Once this is successfully accomplished, the individual is considered to be board-certified in both internal medicine and rheumatology. It is preferable that all of this training has taken place at one of the top medical university programs in the United States or elsewhere in the world. I am going through this in some detail because I want you to understand the background and qualifications of the specific physician you need to seek out. You need to find yourself a rheumatologist, because when it comes to arthritis rheumatologists do it better.

The Value of a Rheumatologist

There are over one hundred different rheumatic diseases. Some of these confine their damage primarily to the joints while others may involve internal organs as well. The most common form of arthritis, osteoarthritis (degenerative arthritis), with its typical involvement of the end joints and middle joints of the hands is a more straightforward diagnosis. If you have a very mild form of osteoarthritis, then your primary care physician may be able to handle your treatment successfully. When it comes to a more complicated rheumatic condition such as systemic lupus erythematosus, with its multiple presentations and with its complicated laboratory findings, then a rheumatologist is essential to properly sort things out. Some primary care physicians are very familiar with osteoarthritis and rheumatoid arthritis, but are not as savvy when it comes to the less common forms of arthritis. Diagnostic possibilities become more complex, because often these diseases may mimic one another thus clouding the proper diagnosis. Chondrocalcinosis with the depositing of calcium pyrophosphate crystals in the cartilage may lead to pseudogout episodes, which may be difficult to differentiate from gout. Psoriasis of the skin may have an associated form of arthritis called psoriatic arthritis, which can sometimes imitate the findings in rheumatoid arthritis. Psoriatic arthritis can occasionally manifest itself with large painful sausage-shaped toes, but this needs to be distinguished from another condition called Reiter's syndrome where similar changes in the toes can occur.

Some patients may start off with signs and symptoms that are fairly typical for rheumatoid arthritis, but then later in the course of their illness start complaining of lupus-related problems. These patients may have a rheumatoid arthritis-systemic lupus erythematosus overlap syndrome sometimes referred to as "rhupus." This would usually be confusing to a primary care physician and not normally within their level of expertise.

Some people, who are quite ill, will present to the doctor with symptoms and laboratory findings that indicate the involvement of multiple internal organs in the body. The diagnostic work-up that is required in this setting is extremely elaborate and complex and calls forth all of the knowledge gleaned from the years of university training in rheumatology. If a diagnosis of systemic (involvement of multiple systems in the body) vasculitis (inflammation of the blood vessel walls) can be made accurately and quickly, then this may actually end up being life-saving.

I would guess that most of you have experienced some type of muscular pain in your life. In a person over the age of sixty-five, however, muscular symptoms in the upper arms and thighs could represent a disorder called polymyalgia rheumatica. It can sometimes be a subtle disorder, but one that is very familiar to a rheumatologist. Unfortunately, it can be associated with another condition called temporal arteritis or giant cell arteritis. This form of vasculitis can potentially lead to sudden loss of vision or a stroke, so that it is imperative that this entity be properly diagnosed with prompt treatment instituted. A delay in diagnosis because you are not under the care of a rheumatologist could cost you your eyesight if you go untreated.

Other patients with muscular symptoms may be experiencing severe weakness. It may be difficult to brush or wash one's hair. Stepping up on a curb or being able to lift oneself out of a chair may become difficult or impossible. A rheumatologist can sort out the history, the physical findings on an examination, and the laboratory results to conclude that this is from an actual autoimmune assault on the muscles called polymyositis. Very potent medicines may need to be started to control this process and this requires considerable expertise to do it correctly and well.

Some patients have muscular pain, which seems to involve all of the muscles of their body. Often, exacerbations occur with changes in the weather or even after stress or emotional problems. Patients may have multiple tender areas overlying many muscles in the neck, upper back, and lower back, and yet the laboratory testing is unrevealing. These patients may be experiencing fibromyalgia syndrome, a condition that is best diagnosed and treated by rheumatologists.

Fibromyalgia is controversial, in part, because physicians do not understand it well and because no specific lab test makes it readily diagnosable. Some of you may have previously seen a television program focusing on fibromyalgia, which pitted a nationally renowned rheumatologist and fibromyalgia expert with a group of neurologists. The neurologists, in their frustration over not being able to easily understand this disorder, decided by a show of hands to vote fibromyalgia out of existence. It would be as if rheumatologists voted to do away with the diagnosis of multiple sclerosis or Parkinson's disease. At some point in time, the symptoms and signs of these neurological diseases also must have mystified physicians, until sufficient medical knowledge was able to explain what these patients were experiencing.

New information is being discovered each year that helps to

shed more light on the subject of fibromyalgia. For example, there is evidence that a compound called substance P may be present in increased amounts in the spinal fluid of some patients with this condition. This may be associated with an increased sensitivity to touch and to painful stimuli applied to the muscular tissues of the body. It may take many years before we totally understand this disorder, but in the meantime rheumatologists remain at the forefront of the clinical research and advances in treatment of fibromyalgia. Out of ignorance, physicians will imply or even actually state to patients that they think the problem is "all in the patient's head," i.e., a psychiatric problem. Although psychological factors may sometimes play a role in this condition, it is a disservice to the patient to imply that what they are experiencing is imagined. Instead, we should respect the patient's complaints and realize that as physicians we may be limited in our understanding of a condition like fibromyalgia by our own ignorance. A fibromyalgia patient will find that a rheumatologist will be the most sympathetic of all physicians regarding their complaints. The rheumatology specialist will take the most interest in putting together a multi-pronged approach to treatment of the patient, rather than dismissing him as simply being a depressed or anxious individual.

Thus, the rheumatologist is the doctor with the most knowledge of these many musculo-skeletal disorders and is uniquely qualified to provide you with an accurate diagnosis. Musculo-skeletal conditions include problems related to the bones and joints, as well as the muscles, tendons, and ligaments. Since there are over one hundred types of rheumatic diseases, it is essential that the right questions be posed to you during your initial history obtained in the doctor's office. Many rheumatologists even have thoughtfully and carefully devised medical history forms to assist in the collection of this important information. If some of these subtle points in your history are not brought out by proper inquiry, then the final diagnosis may not be correct. It is the rheumatologist, who by constantly reading about these disorders and keeping up with the new medical literature is best able to glean from your story what is important and to put the puzzle parts together.

A Rheumatologist is also an Internist

Once an elaborate and detailed history has been obtained, you will undergo a complete physical examination. Since rheumatologists are also board-certified in internal medicine, all of your organ systems will be checked out. The rheumatologist is educated regarding major diseases, such as diabetes mellitus, thyroid disease, hypertension and heart disease, and different types of cancer. This enables the rheumatology specialist to decide which of your complaints is a consequence of another medical illness and which is due to a separate rheumatologic disorder. In addition to a basic physical examination, you will also undergo a musculo-skeletal exam. The doctor will examine each of the joints of your body, looking for any swelling or tenderness. Thickening of the lining of a joint (called synovitis due to thickening of the synovial lining) may be quite subtle and easy to miss by an untrained observer. Yet, it is the finding of synovitis that is the hallmark of rheumatoid arthritis and would be essential to note in order to properly make this diagnosis. A rheumatologist also puts each joint through its normal range of motion. If movement is limited, then it needs to be noted and reasons for this deficit sought out. If a joint has a crunchy or cracking feeling as it is moved (crepitation), then this may suggest underlying structural damage, such as may be seen in degenerative arthritis (osteoarthritis). If the patient has accumulated an excess amount of fluid in a joint such as the knee, then a rheumatologist is able to discover this, even when the amount may be small and possibly overlooked. This may be important, however, in affording the physician an opportunity to drain this fluid and then submit the liquid for a complete and careful analysis. An examination for crystals under a special polarizing microscope will facilitate the diagnosis of gout or pseudogout immediately after the joint has been aspirated. In my twenty-five plus years of rheumatologic practice, I have seen innumerable patients who were told that they had gout, but never had been accurately and correctly diagnosed with this disease by crystal analysis of a joint fluid sample. In some of these cases, unnecessary medications had been erroneously started on the basis of a wrong diagnosis.

The Rheumatologist as Diagnostician

Once the history and proper physical examination have been completed, the rheumatologist's thought processes are functioning at full throttle. Based on these findings, the rheumatologist, in most cases, already has a fairly good idea of what your problem is. In other, more mysterious situations, the hunt is on to ferret out a correct diagnosis. The rheumatologist will put together a list of laboratory tests that are essential to arrive at the proper diagnosis. Included in the list should also be other tests that are related to the safety of medications that will be initiated. These will include liver and kidney blood tests. The rheumatologist may start with an initial panel of tests and only add more sophisticated studies at a subsequent visit if the first tests come back with an abnormal reading. In some cases, such as in an individual with lateral epicondylitis (tennis elbow), only the most basic tests are required regarding the use of anti-inflammatory medicines. A less knowledgeable physician will often order a much larger array of tests because of their uncertainty about the diagnosis, even after a history and exam. This adds further expense to the cost of your care that could have been avoided by a specialist who already understood what was going on, without resorting to lab or x-rays that were really unnecessary.

I see a fair number of patients each year in consultation, for example, due to the finding of a positive anti-nuclear antibody (ANA) in their blood. The primary care physician may have received a report about a patient's positive ANA result, but may be uncertain as to its significance. By the time the patient sees me, they are already in a state of panic after being told by their primary doctor that they may have lupus. Their anxiety will only be relieved when subsequent evaluation by me refutes this diagnosis. Many physicians, who are not trained in rheumatology, have been educated to equate a positive ANA with the diagnosis of lupus. There are, however, many other explanations for a positive test. Medications, for example, can trigger a positive result. The most common culprits include Isoniazid (INH) used to treat tuberculosis, Procainamide used to treat heart rhythm disturbances, Hydralazine for high blood pressure, and Dilantin utilized as a treatment for seizures. Once these medications are discontinued, the ANA may subsequently revert to "negative" or normal. Aging alone can contribute to a positive ANA (low titer). Thyroid disorders, such as Hashimoto's thyroiditis, that lead to hypothyroidism (under-active thyroid), or Grave's disease with hyperthyroidism, may be associated with a positive ANA. Liver diseases, including chronic active hepatitis, may trigger a positive ANA blood test. An abnormal ANA test may also be found in rheumatoid arthritis, Sjogren's syndrome, polymyositis, scleroderma, and other rheumatologic conditions without the presence of systemic lupus erythematosus. A rheumatologist is the best-trained physician to clarify the significance of an abnormality of the anti-nuclear antibody test and put it in its proper context. Many a patient has left my office tremendously relieved when I had clarified an abnormal report and put their mind at ease that in their case it held no great significance.

The ability to know which tests to order regarding joint and muscular complaints, and then how to interpret the results correctly, takes special training. Many of these newer tests are complicated and require a sophisticated knowledge of serologic tests as they pertain to rheumatic diseases. A positive rheumatoid factor, for example, is not equivalent to having rheumatoid arthritis. A patient still needs to manifest synovitis in multiple joints (often in a symmetrical distribution in the body) over a period of several months. Chronic infections, pulmonary fibrosis, aging, and other situations may also be associated with a positive rheumatoid factor antibody titer.

Another very frequent reason that people are sent to see me is for an abnormal sedimentation rate (ESR) on lab testing. This is a test done to screen for inflammation in the body, but the problem is that it is very non-specific. Thus, if you have chronic allergies with sinus problems, your sedimentation rate is likely to be at least mildly elevated. Very high sedimentation rates are more worrisome and may be associated with active rheumatoid arthritis, polymyalgia rheumatica, aggressive involvement with lupus, active vasculitis, or other serious rheumatic diseases. It may also be associated with other significant medical conditions, such as cancer or severe infections. On the other hand, a normal ESR is seen in fibromyalgia syndrome. Rheumatologists, therefore, are one of the key types of physicians called upon to interpret an abnormal ESR, along with hematologists/oncologists, and infectious diseases specialists among others.

Rheumatologists are Experts in the Diagnosis and Treatment of Osteoporosis

Rheumatologists also have a particular interest in the evaluation and treatment of osteoporosis. This condition is not a form of arthritis. It is a type of metabolic bone disease with decreased bone density and associated architectural changes leading to more fragile bone and the potential for fractures. Nowadays, most rheumatologists have a dual energy x-ray absorptiometry (DEXA) machine in their offices in order to properly measure the density of the bones of the lumbar spine and the femur (hip). These are the two most critical areas to measure in order to decide on whether a patient needs specific treatment for osteoporosis. Since diseases such as rheumatoid arthritis and systemic lupus erythematosus are more frequently seen in women, rheumatologists tend to see a predominantly female adult population. It is, therefore, logical for rheumatologists to also be assessing for osteoporotic changes in bone, which occur more commonly in females. Also inflammatory joint diseases like rheumatoid arthritis are associated with osteoporotic changes in bone. Some of this may be as a result of inactivity and lack of exercise due to the disease, but newer research has also demonstrated a connection with increased amounts of interleukin-1 found in RA. Interleukin-1 (IL-1) contributes not only to the inflammation in the synovial lining of the joints, but also to the breakdown of cartilage and the osteoporosis found in this condition. In rheumatoid arthritis and a number of other rheumatic disorders, corticosteroids may be required as temporary measures to control the activity of the disease. Unfortunately, one of the side effects of prolonged or high dose steroid therapy is the development of steroid-induced osteoporosis. Rheumatologists, therefore, have yet another reason to closely monitor these individuals for any osteoporotic changes. The earlier that treatment can be instituted and detrimental medicine eliminated, the more likely it is that the patient may avoid future fractures and the disability they can cause.

Rheumatologists and Your X-Rays

X-rays are often an essential part of an initial rheumatologic evaluation and rheumatologists are specially trained to read them. There are a number of things on joint films that are particularly important. One of the most critical assessments is to check for any evidence of joint space narrowing. When an individual complains of knee pain, it is helpful to know whether the patient still has adequate joint space left between the thigh bone (femur) and the main leg bone (tibia). If these bones are touching, then this has implications regarding what treatment options are available. Another factor worth evaluating is whether there are any erosions of bone at the joints themselves. In rheumatoid arthritis, the presence of erosive disease of the bone is a forerunner of deformities in the joints. Multiple erosions may be associated with more aggressive forms of rheumatoid arthritis. These patients are candidates for the newer forms of treatment, including biologic therapies and disease modifying anti-rheumatic drugs (DMARDs). These will be discussed in more detail in Step 5. Another group of patients with low back pain may have spinal x-rays that show evidence of disc space narrowing, collapse of the vertebrae themselves, arthritic spurs, and other abnormalities. There are innumerable other x-ray abnormalities associated with rheumatic diseases, but suffice it to say that a rheumatologist is best able to tell you whether or not obtaining an x-ray might help in your diagnosis or aid in deciding on the best course of treatment for your condition.

The Rheumatologist and Your Treatment Plan

When it comes to treatment recommendations for your rheumatic disorder, the rheumatologist once again is uniquely qualified to direct you in the proper direction. All too frequently, arthritis patients arriving for their first consultation with me have previously been treated by their primary care physician with non-steroidal anti-inflammatory drugs (NSAIDs), but this has been the full extent of their therapy. The field of rheumatology has blossomed in the 1990s with the advent of new or combination DMARD therapy, and then more recently with the revolutionary development of targeted biologic therapies. These treatments will be addressed in Steps 4 and 5 of our 12 step approach to taking back control of your arthritis.

Rheumatologists are quite skilled at combining multiple different categories of medications, along with the use of injections, adjunctive physical therapy, and exercise. A good illustration of this is in the treatment of fibromyalgia patients. Rheumatologists often need to prescribe a pain medicine, a muscle relaxant, an anti-depressant, a sleeping pill, and sometimes an NSAID to adequately treat a fibromyalgia patient suffering with significant muscular spasm and pain. Massage and physical therapy may need to be added to the mix. Then eventually when the patient is doing better, an exercise program is recommended to help the patient stretch and condition the muscles as part of a long-term program.

The treatment of rheumatoid arthritis has now gotten more complicated with the advent of new therapies. At the onset, a rheumatologist needs to judge how aggressive treatment needs to be. In mild disease, it may be sufficient to start with an NSAID combined with low dosages of tapering corticosteroids and a milder DMARD such as Plaquenil (hydroxy-chloroquine). In more severe cases, this would be inadequate. Methotrexate, along with an NSAID, subsequently followed by the addition of one of the biologics may be more appropriate. Similar to the hematologist/oncologist who adjusts various combinations of chemotherapeutic agents, the rheumatologist now juggles these various medications to design the perfect therapeutic "cocktail" for that individual.

Knowing When and How to Order Physical Therapy

Many rheumatologic practices have their own physical therapy modalities present in the office. Patients may be treated with ultrasound, electrical stimulation of the muscles, hydrocollator packs (hot packs) or paraffin, and massage to provide additional relief to tight and painful muscles. In the case of a patient, who has cervical disc disease with nerve root pain radiating down the arm, the use of intermittent traction with a machine that stretches the neck may be extremely beneficial. Physical therapists may be called upon to teach the patient appropriate exercises to strengthen the tissues surrounding a joint. Patients are given instructions for a home program that includes stretching, strengthening, and conditioning. Knowing when to arrange for this type of adjunctive treatment in combination with medical therapy is part of the "art" of practicing rheumatology.

Knowing When and How to Inject

Part of this "art" certainly includes the judicious injections of medications into the joints, muscles, and other soft tissues of the body. This is a skill that is taught during the doctor's rheumatology fellowship training. A knowledgeable rheumatologist will be able to decide whether it is more appropriate to treat your disorder with adjustments of the doses or types of medication you are taking, versus injecting a particular joint. In osteoarthritis of the knee, injections of viscosupplements are now an important additional treatment option. The two most commonly utilized materials, Synvisc and Hyalgan, are injected once a week for three weeks. It is essential that these viscous substances be injected into the joint and not just adjacent to the joint. A higher degree of skill with joint injections is necessary to make sure that the needle is within the joint before injecting. In a patient with severe narrowing under the knee cap (patella), it may be necessary to inject the knee with the patient in the non-standard seated position. A rheumatologist has the special training to properly accomplish this.

There are other more difficult injections that almost always require the expertise of a rheumatologist or orthopedic surgeon.

These include injections in the first carpal metacarpal joint at the base of the thumb, in the tissues adjacent to the flexor tendons of the hand (to relieve "trigger" finger), in the elbow and shoulder joints, and in the heel for plantar fasciitis and heel spurs, along with a number of other locations. Rheumatologists are also skilled at injecting either a mixture of xylocaine and steroids, or just xylocaine alone in areas of tenderness overlying muscles. This may be utilized as part of the treatment of patients with tender points ("trigger points") in fibromyalgia syndrome.

Why Outcomes with Rheumatologists are Better

In outcome studies dealing with differences in the consequences of treatment by primary care physicians versus rheumatologists in the treatment of rheumatic diseases, results have shown significant benefit in being under the care of a rheumatologist. In osteoarthritis, this difference is largely accounted for by the additional use of injections and physical therapy by rheumatologists, whereas primary care physicians seem to rely principally on medications. As the treatment of rheumatoid arthritis becomes more complex, the gap in outcomes between rheumatologists and doctors without special training should widen further. More complicated rheumatologic problems, such as systemic vasculitis or systemic lupus erythematosus, demand the special knowledge of a rheumatologist familiar with treatment of these potentially life-threatening conditions.

Unfortunately, I am aware of situations where primary care doctors would not grant rheumatic disease patients referrals for specialty care. Some of these patients were actually misdiagnosed and then given inappropriate treatment for their disease. For example, patients were told that they had rheumatoid arthritis when in fact they had osteoarthritis. They were then prescribed drugs designed for the treatment of rheumatoid arthritis, which do not work in osteoarthritis. These patients were exposed to potential toxicities of these medications unnecessarily.

Before the days of managed care, there was rarely an incident where patients with significant rheumatologic problems were not appropriately referred to a rheumatologist, but that has changed with the advent of HMOs. There are still managed care plans that include financial incentives for the primary care physician not to refer the patient to a specialist. In other words, at the end of the year, a primary care physician may earn more money if he or she does not refer the patient for consultation or perform blood tests or x-rays. Usually the patient is completely unaware of this financial arrangement. To me this is a totally unethical situation. The patient generally assumes that their physician would recommend the best treatment available for their condition. Any contractual arrangements that potentially jeopardize the patient should be fully disclosed. In this terribly ill conceived situation, the primary care physician has pitted his or her own financial gain versus the patient's health. When one considers the allure of money, you can guess who loses out. If a primary care physician adamantly refuses to refer you to a rheumatologist, then you have a few options. You can try switching to a different primary care physician who is willing to place your health above any personal financial concerns. If this does not work, then you may need to switch to a different health plan that has a more liberal attitude towards patients seeing specialists. Some HMOs have changed their rules so that patients can now make appointments with specialists on their own without going through a lot of bureaucratic hassle.

In the patient with inflammatory arthritis, who is not referred to a rheumatologist in a timely manner, there are other consequences to consider. Patients with rheumatoid arthritis may develop erosions within months following the onset of this disease. Rheumatologists are now trained to look for these erosions and start aggressive therapy immediately once these are discovered.

Otherwise, these patients may wind up with advanced destructive disease complicated by deformities. If a primary care doctor is not aware of this risk and continues to treat with NSAIDs alone, the patient will suffer the consequences. You need to realize that many of these primary care physicians may have only received a few weeks of education in medical school concerning the rheumatic diseases, so that their knowledge is often superficial at best. Certainly they may get additional post-graduate education from medical journals, at seminars, or national meetings, but their training is usually neither rigorous nor comprehensive. Also it is virtually impossible for a primary care physician to keep up completely with every single medical sub-specialty. It is demanding enough for the specialist himself to just remain current with his or her own single specialty.

Some primary care physicians may be familiar with some of the new, more advanced treatments in the rheumatic illnesses. As a result of this, they may start the patient on these therapies, some of which may have toxic reactions. The problem is that often they are not familiar with all of the side effects of these treatments and sometimes do not know how to properly monitor for these toxicities. This is a form of "medical Russian roulette." Some patients will luck out and not have significant problems with these therapies, but others may develop organ damage or even fatal complications. This is particularly sad if the patient has been started on the wrong medication following an incorrect diagnosis.

In addition to a patient obtaining an accurate diagnosis and being properly monitored on medications, another important reason to be under the care of a rheumatologist has to do with knowing when it is time for you to be referred to an orthopedic surgeon for joint replacement surgery. Over the years, I have had patients consult with me as to whether they should proceed with a joint replacement after being told by another physician that they needed this surgery. In the knee or hip, a joint replacement is often required when the patient has completely lost the cartilage and is "bone on bone." On occasion, when I review their x-rays, I am stunned to find a fairly normal joint space still present. Clearly this patient has not exhausted all of his or her options for continued conservative (non-surgical) care. Although this deceit disturbs me, it should not really be all that surprising. A surgeon makes his or her major money by operating, not by prescribing NSAIDs. They are trained to think mainly in terms of a surgical approach to the treatment of arthritic conditions, although they also utilize medications and injections. Thankfully, most of the orthopedic surgeons I work with are ethical and will only recommend surgery as a last resort after all conservative treatment has failed. If a patient is under the principal care of a rheumatologist, then he or she can talk it over and decide if the time has come to proceed with surgery. It is preferable to discuss the best mode of treatment with a doctor, who does not have any financial benefits for recommending surgery earlier than necessary. In the case of osteoarthritis of the knee, patients should have failed to respond to oral medication, intra-articular steroid injections, as well as a trial of viscosupplementation injections before surgery is recommended.

Being Sensitive to Your Pain

Rheumatologists are almost always treating patients who are in significant pain. Thus, they are very sensitive to the pain medication (analgesic) requirements of their patients. Clearly, if they are not successful in dealing with their patients' discomfort, then they will not have much of a practice. As a group, rheumatologists tend to be very sympathetic and are always interested in trying new and improved pain medications to better control their patients symptoms. In Step 3, I will discuss the need to take back control of your pain and will give you a lot of information about different medications that may help you.

Rheumatologists also understand how to combine anti-depressant medications with the pain medicines to reduce pain further.

It should be apparent to you by now that the rheumatologist is the physician best suited to take care of your rheumatic condition. The rheumatologist has the knowledge, training, and experience to properly diagnose and treat your arthritis or other rheumatic condition. The rheumatology specialist is the doctor who is most knowledgeable about the benefits and risks of all of the treatment options available. The rheumatologist possesses the wisdom to know when to combine multiple medications in conjunction with other types of treatment such as physical therapy and joint injections. If you are going to take back control of your arthritis in these twelve steps, then you must not only find yourself a doctor who you can communicate with and trust, but you also need to hook up with the very best rheumatologist in your area.

Key Points in Finding a Rheumatologist:

1. If you have a significant form of arthritis or other rheumatic condition, find yourself the best rheumatologist in your vicinity.

2. If you are in an HMO and are experiencing difficulty obtaining a referral to see a rheumatologist, you should consider changing your primary care physician or even changing to a different health plan that will allow you the specialty care that you need.

3. Do not allow yourself to be trapped by your health insurance into being treated by a primary care physician, who lacks the special training and experience to treat significant rheumatic disorders optimally.

4. Ask physicians, family, friends, and other rheumatic disease patients for their recommendation about a rheumatologist in your region.

5. Find a rheumatologist who is preferably board-certified in both internal medicine and rheumatology and has been trained at a major university medical center.

6. If you are considering joint replacement surgery, make certain that your rheumatologist has reviewed your medical condition and your x-rays, and then concurs. Also you should be convinced that you have exhausted all conservative medical treatments before proceeding with surgery.

Step 3: Take Back Control of Your Pain

Telltale Signs That Your Pain Is Not Adequately Controlled:

- Even with your medication, your pain is never completely relieved.

- Your pain awakens you out of your sleep at night.

- Your pain prevents you from doing even menial tasks at home.

- Your pain makes it impossible for you to function in any work situation.

- The constant pain is making you miserable and depressed.

- The pain is making you excessively irritable and anxious.

- The pain is affecting your interpersonal relationships in your marriage, family, or work setting.

- You feel like your doctor doesn't really believe you when you explain how much pain you are experiencing.

- The pain medicines help to a certain degree, but you are having side effects, which force you to take less medicine.

- The pain prevents you from having pleasurable sexual activity with your spouse or partner.

- You are afraid of becoming addicted to the pain medicines so you do not take them as prescribed by your doctor.

Don't Let Your Pain Ruin Your Life

Most of the patients who come to see me in my office do so because they are in pain. Many of them may have tried to self-medicate with over-the-counter preparations. Some have been to their primary care physician, but the medicine they were given was not strong enough to control their pain. Others have actually tried to ignore the problem and the pain, but over time it has gradually worsened to the point where they realized that they needed help.

Pain can completely dominate your life if you allow it to do so. You can awaken each morning in pain, struggle with pain throughout your waking hours, and then try to fall asleep at night in spite of your pain. Pain can interfere with your ability to earn a living. It can change your personality and make you hyperirritable or depressed. This, in turn, can change your relationship with your spouse, your children, your friends, or co-workers. Pain can destroy all of the pleasure that you previously had in your life, including the joy you had from your loved ones, your hobbies, and even your sexual activity. Thus, if your pain is permitted to continue unabated, it can slowly but surely ruin your life.

Some Rheumatic Causes of Pain

The sources of the pain from musculo-skeletal diseases are numerous. The lining of the joints, called the synovium, has nerve endings present. When the synovium becomes significantly inflamed, as it does in rheumatoid arthritis and other forms of inflammatory arthritis, then the patient may feel intense pain in the involved joint. In osteoarthritis, which is synonymous with degenerative arthritis, the primary problem is in the cartilage, which deteriorates over time. There also may be a mild degree of inflammation present which could cause the nerve endings in the synovium to be irritated. There are no nerve endings in the cartilage itself, however. As the cartilage disintegrates, eventually there is no significant cartilaginous covering over the ends of the bones. This results in direct bony contact ("bone on bone").

Muscles may also become painful. They have nerve endings present which can be irritated if the muscle is overstretched or strained. If a muscle is persistently in spasm, it may outstrip the body's ability to supply the muscle fibers with oxygen. Muscles that are not getting sufficient oxygen can be a source of pain.

There are a number of reasons for pain in the neck and back. Discs act as a cushion or shock absorber between the bones of the spine (vertebra). These discs may rupture and put pressure on the spinal cord or the nerve roots that exit out to your extremities. This may produce a radiating type pain down the arm or leg, sometimes associated with numbness, tingling, or burning. There are joints in the spine itself and these can develop osteoarthritis. These joints can undergo the same type of joint space narrowing and bony contact that we see in the peripheral joints of the body. Spurs (osteophytes) may form in this situation and exert pressure on important nerves in the spinal area. This is another source of potential spinal pain or radiating pain into the limbs. When you go to the doctor and complain of pain in your spine or limbs, it is critical that your physician have the ability to recognize and differentiate amongst these different types and sources of pain.

Assessing Pain

Your doctor should also be in the habit of quantifying the severity of your pain, not just on your first visit, but also on each and every subsequent visit. If he or she is not doing this, then you may want to consider switching to someone who is more focused on assessing your degree of pain and then doing something about it. New hospital guidelines have recently been established, which make it a requirement for your pain to be assessed each day that you are in the hospital. Along with the nurses needing to check your vital signs including your pulse, temperature, and blood pressure, they are now also obligated to assess your level of pain. This is easily accomplished by what is called a visual analog scale for pain. A horizontal line on a piece of paper is divided into equal sections and numbered from zero to ten from left to right. The patient is then asked to draw a vertical line through the horizontal line to indicate their level of pain, with zero meaning no pain whatsoever and ten signifying the worst pain possible. Monitoring your level of pain can indicate to the physician whether he or she is adequately controlling your pain or not.

Doctors Differ in their Treatment of Pain

You will find physicians, unfortunately, who are very reluctant to prescribe pain medicines. One would suspect that these doctors had never experienced severe and incapacitating pain firsthand in their own lives. One would think that any prior personal encounter would have sensitized them to the whole issue of adequate pain management. Some doctors have been "burned" in the past and now are not very trusting. They worry about being manipulated by individuals who insist on stronger narcotics for treatment. A number of prior studies have shown that doctors do tend to under treat pain symptoms. This is even more of a problem if they lack the objective support on x-rays or laboratory testing to justify the need for more potent drugs. Fibromyalgia syndrome is a painful musculo-skeletal condition, which lacks objective parameters such as abnormal laboratory results. Fibromyalgia patients, however, often complain bitterly about the constant and severe nature of their widespread pain. In this situation the rheumatologist, who is most familiar with this condition, is probably best suited to judge whether the patient's complaints are valid and then treat them adequately.

Basic Information about Pain Medicines

Pain medications as a group are referred to as analgesics. The non-steroidal anti-inflammatory medicines (NSAIDs), which I will discuss in the next chapter, also afford some degree of pain relief (analgesia) even if they are being prescribed primarily to control joint inflammation. In some situations, therefore, it is possible to use an NSAID and not require an additional pain medicine (analgesic). When NSAIDs are used in doses below those required to achieve an anti-inflammatory effect, any benefit comes just from their pain-relieving qualities. For example, ibuprofen has anti-inflammatory effects when the dose exceeds 1600 mg on a daily and regular basis. Over-the-counter forms of ibuprofen, including Advil, Nuprin, and Mediprin contain 200 mg of medication in each tablet. If a patient takes four to six tablets of these preparations per day, this will not be an anti-inflammatory dose, but may provide some pain relief.

Every medicine, whether it is an anti-inflammatory medicine, an analgesic drug, or any other type of medication has a generic name. It is also then marketed by the pharmaceutical company under a brand name. It should not astound you that the brand names chosen by the pharmaceutical companies often are meant to be highly suggestive of being beneficial to you. When it comes to pain medication names, there is Norco (hydrocodone plus acetaminophen), which certainly sounds similar to the word "narcotic." Ultram (tramadol) is a different pain medication that is close to the word "ultra" which might possibly imply that it could be "ultra-effective" or "ultra-beneficial." The generic forms of these tablets are supposed to be equivalent to the brand name drugs, and are, of course, a whole lot cheaper. Yet, I have a number of patients who insist on my writing for "brand name only" claiming that they can tell a significant difference between the brand name and the generic substitute. It is still unclear to me whether their claims are valid or not. Therefore, I would recommend that you simply need to find out on your own if the less expensive generic pain pill is adequate for you and equivalent to the brand name medication or not.

Table 3.1
Commonly Prescribed Pain Medications (Analgesics)

Generic Name of Medication	Brand Name of Medication
Acetaminophen	Tylenol
Acetaminophen with butalbital and caffeine	Fioricet, Esgic
Propoxyphene	Darvon, Darvon N
Propoxyphene with acetaminophen	Darvocet-N, Darvocet A500
Propoxyphene with aspirin and caffeine	Darvon compound
Tramadol	Ultram
Tramadol with acetaminophen	Ultracet
Acetaminophen with codeine	Tylenol No. 3, Tylenol No. 4
Pentazocine	Talwin NX
Hydrocodone with acetaminophen	Vicodin, Zydone, Norco, Lortabs, Lorcet
Hydrocodone with ibuprofen	Vicoprofen
Oxycodone	Roxicodone
Oxycodone with aspirin	Percodan
Oxycodone with acetaminophen	Percocet, Tylox, Roxicet
Slow release oxycodone	Oxycontin
Fentanyl patch	Duragesic patch
Morphine sulfate	MS Contin, MSIR. Kadian, Avinza

An Overview of Pain Medicines

There is a certain "pecking order" of pain medication, ranging from acetaminophen as a mild painkiller, up to the very strongest narcotics like morphine.

Acetaminophen is known to most people under its brand name of Tylenol. In spite of the tragedy years ago with the tampering of Tylenol containers and deaths from cyanide, the drug still remains popular. Regular Strength Tylenol contains 325 mg of acetaminophen, Extra Strength Tylenol has 500 mg, and Arthritis Strength Tylenol has 650 mg. Some of you are reluctant to take Tylenol because you are fearful about liver and kidney side effects. Much of that concern arose from studies in Europe with individuals who far exceeded the recommended dosages. Some of the deaths that occurred due to liver disease were in people who were imbibing a great deal of alcohol while on acetamenophen.

Acetaminophen (Tylenlol) appears safe to take if you do not exceed a total of more than four grams (4000 mg) in a twenty-four hour period. Eight Extra Strength Tylenol would come out to exactly 4000 mg per day since each one has 500 mg in it. Eight Arthritis Strength Tylenol, on the other hand, would exceed this limit (8 X 650 mg). Six Arthritis Strength Tylenol per day would put you back safely within the recommended dose limit. In calculating your total dosage it is essential that you also include other quantities of acetaminophen that may be mixed in with other over-the-counter or prescription medicines as well. Many patients are unaware that their Darvocet N, Vicodin, or Lortab pain tablets also contain acetaminophen. The quantity of acetaminophen present in these tablets taken each day needs to be subtracted from the 4000 mg total in order to calculate whether you are safely within the recommended dose.

If acetaminophen (Tylenol) is ineffective in completely controlling your pain, then the next step up on the analgesic ladder may be to try propoxyphene napsylate (Darvon), which is a mild narcotic. There are a number of different formulations of this analgesic, including Darvon compound, which combines aspirin with 65 mg of propoxyphene. Darvocet N 100 has been used to combat pain for many years. It contains 100 mg of propoxyphene along with 650 mg of acetaminophen. If a patient takes more than six of these tablets per day, this would exceed the 4000 mg limit on acetaminophen. In recent years, one way to get around this was to prescribe a pure form of propoxyphene called Darvon N 100, which contains 100 mg of the pain medication alone without any acetaminophen. Patients would just add any additional acetaminophen as needed to this, while making sure that they did not go over the 4000 mg level. A new formulation of propoxyphene, however, may simplify things for some arthritis sufferers. Darvocet A500 is a combination of propoxyphene 100 mg and acetaminophen 500 mg. Therefore, even if patients take eight of these tablets per day they will still be within the 4000 mg window on acetaminophen. With any of these different formulations of propoxyphene, side effects may include constipation, nausea, vomiting, dizziness, or sedation. These problems may actually be encountered with any of the narcotic analgesic type medications.

Another medicine that offers a fairly similar degree of pain relief is tramadol (Ultram). It should not be used in patients who have a history of seizures. It also has the potential to aggravate any underlying liver or kidney problems and, therefore, should be used cautiously or even avoided in patients with these problems. It is usually best to start off slowly with 50 mg tablets taken up to four times a day, and then only gradually advance up to 100 mg four times daily if absolutely necessary. Some patients may experience central nervous system side effects with headaches or dizziness secondary to this medicine. A new formulation of Ultram called Ultracet contains 37.5 mg of tramadol with 325 mg of acetaminophen in a single tablet. This is often given on a four times a day basis. It has the same side effect profile and concerns associated with Ultram itself.

Codeine can be prescribed by itself, but is more commonly taken in combination with acetaminophen. Tylenol number three (Tylenol

No. 3) contains 30 mg of codeine per tablet, whereas Tylenol number four (Tylenol No. 4) has 60 mg of codeine. Some people are allergic to codeine as manifested by itching of the skin or an actual rash, while others have central nervous side effects, or nausea and vomiting. Interestingly, some people who are unable to tolerate codeine can take synthetic forms of hydrocodone without similar reactions.

Pain relief may be obtained from tablets that contain a barbiturate with acetaminophen. Fioricet and Esgic combine the barbiturate butalbital with acetaminophen and caffeine. Fiorinal has aspirin present in it (instead of acetaminophen) along with the butalbital and caffeine. These compounds may even be combined with 30 mg of codeine to make them even more potent. This group of pain medicines is most commonly used for severe headaches, but I have sometimes prescribed them for patients in pain who were intolerant of Darvon or hydrocodone preparations.

Another alternative for the treatment of moderate pain is talacen (Talwin or Talwin NX). Originally when it was first released, it was promoted as a less addicting painkiller, but this has proven to be overstated. The Talwin NX actually contains a narcotic antagonist, naloxone, in the tablet. If the tablet is crushed in an attempt to abuse it by injecting it intravenously, the naloxone will prevent the "high" that one might get after receiving a sudden burst of a significant amount of talacen alone. Central nervous system side effects may occur. Occasionally patients have described feeling "spaced out" and feel as though they have "tripped out" after taking Talwin.

There are a number of different pharmaceutical companies that make a stronger pain medicine called hydrocodone. It is produced under various brand names including Vicodin, Zydone, Norco, Lortabs, and Lorcet. This is usually prescribed as 5 mg, 7.5 mg, or 10 mg tablets up to four times a day. It is most commonly given in combination with differing quantities of acetaminophen. Once again it is important to calculate the total amount of acetaminophen consumed per day even when combined with hydrocodone and make certain that it does not exceed the 4000 mg limit. In fact, Norco was marketed on the basis that it contained a lower amount of acetaminophen in each tablet (325 mg). This was less than what was available at the time in the other formulations combining hydrocodone and acetaminophen. Extra Strength Vicodin combines 7.5 mg of hydrocodone with 750 mg of acetaminophen. If a patient were to take two tablets four times a day, then he or she would be receiving an excessive amount of acetaminophen. Since hydrocodone is stronger than the medicines we have discussed earlier, it tends to cause more problems with constipation. Stronger narcotics may significantly impair intestinal motility and peristalsis, which is necessary to keep your bowel movements normal.

A slightly different variation on the theme of combining hydrocodone with a second medication is a medicine called Vicoprofen. This tablet consists of 7.5 mg of hydrocodone joined together with the NSAID Ibuprofen 200 mg. This is the same dose of Ibuprofen found in a typical Advil tablet that you could buy over the counter. At this low dose of Ibuprofen, even if this was taken four times a day, there is not any significant anti-inflammatory benefit (more than 1600 mg would be required for that to occur), but rather just the analgesic effect of the Ibuprofen. If you are already taking another NSAID tablet for your arthritis and you are prescribed Vicoprofen for your pain, you will essentially be taking two anti-inflammatory medicines simultaneously. Studies have shown that this does not generally add much additional benefit, but it does result in an increase in your chance of developing side effects such as stomach irritation. If you are not on an existing anti-inflammatory medicine, but have arthritis and would benefit from this type of medicine, then it is probably better to take Ibuprofen separately as a 600 mg or 800 mg tablet three or four times a day with food. Otherwise you will be receiving an inadequate anti-inflammatory dose by taking only the Vicoprofen. You then could supplement your full dose of Ibuprofen with a pure pain pill that is not a combination medicine like Vicoprofen. If you do not need an anti-inflammatory medication, but just pain medication, then Vicoprofen offers the analgesic effect of hydrocodone combined with the pain relieving benefit of Ibuprofen, as opposed to the more commonly prescribed combination of hydrocodone and acetaminophen.

Oxycodone is even one notch higher up on the analgesic ladder than hydrocodone. Percocet, Percodan, Tylox, Roxicodone, and Roxicet are all different brand names of oxycodone. It is also marketed as Oxycodone IR, where the IR stands for immediate release. A slow release formulation was developed by Purdue Pharma and produced under the name Oxycontin. The contin release tablet is a proprietary formulation that they also use in their morphine tablet called MS Contin. Having a tablet that releases medicine slowly and consistently around the clock helps to provide smoother and more constant pain relief. Other analgesic tablets not designed with a slow-release mechanism may only provide shorter-term pain suppression and gradually lose their effect over a number of hours.

Unfortunately, drug abusers have discovered that if they crush the Oxycontin tablet and then chew it, snort it, or inject it intravenously, they can achieve an enormous "high." By crushing the tablet, they are able to bypass the slow release mechanism in the tablet, and instead deliver a huge dose of oxycodone very rapidly. The "high" that they report feeling and the addiction that follows is comparable to heroin. Ramifications from Oxycontin abuse have included thefts and break-ins at pharmacies to try to obtain this drug. Physicians have been drawn into the fray as well. After patients have died as a result of abusing the oxycontin, the prescribing physician has been arrested and charged with manslaughter or even murder. It is not yet clear to me (since I am not privy to the details of each case) whether these doctors had truly done anything wrong or had simply had the misfortune of having one of their patients abuse this medication. This has become a national health concern and even was featured as a news story in a Sunday issue of the *New York Times* magazine section. Once this became a law enforcement issue, the doctors in our clinic elected to stop prescribing the drug. We have instead converted our patients to Oxycodone IR or MS Contin at equivalent doses. Purdue announced that they have begun work on reformulating the tablet so that a narcotic antagonist will be present (similar to the Talwin NX that I described earlier) in combination with the Contin release oxycodone. In that case, if the tablet were crushed, the narcotic antagonist would be released and block the oxycodone from causing a "high." The process of developing and gaining approval of a newly formulated oxycontin tablet could take several years to accomplish.

An alternative way to obtain pain relief, other than by oral tablets, is via a cutaneous patch that delivers medicine to the body through the skin. A Duragesic patch contains the strong narcotic drug fentanyl. Normally, the patch will supply medication for seventy-two hours before it needs to be discarded and replaced with a fresh patch. For individuals who have gastro-intestinal symptoms as a consequence of taking oral pain medication, this offers them a way of receiving potent medicine without having to swallow it. The patches are available in 25, 50, 75, and 100 microgram strengths. If a person needs more than the 100 microgram dose, then the individual will have to combine more than one patch at a time to achieve higher dosages. If the patient has pain that "breaks through" the analgesia afforded by the patch (appropriately called "breakthrough pain"), then the patient may need additional oral medication ("rescue" medication). For example, a patient on a Duragesic patch may still find that he or she needs occasional Darvocet tablets in order to get by.

There are other very potent narcotics that are used to treat extremely severe pain that may occur in cancer patients. These are not typically necessary to control the pain associated with rheumatic diseases. These include Demerol, Dilaudid, methadone, and Stadol. After joint replacement surgery, many patients use patient controlled analgesia (PCA) successfully. Patients are given control of a button to press, which in turn releases Demerol or morphine into their veins. It is devised so that the patient cannot exceed a given dose. This allows the patient to regularly receive narcotic medicine to keep their pain at a reasonable and tolerable level. This is certainly superior to the "old days" when the patient would start ringing their nurse call button when the pain "hit." Then the patient would have to wait in pain until the nurse could prepare an injection of the medication, break away from all of her other responsibilities, and finally come and give the patient a shot.

Some patients may have received a medicine called ketorolac (Toradol) as an intra-muscular injection. This is often given by emergency room physicians to treat a patient's acute pain. It is important to know, however, that this drug is actually part of the NSAID family. It also happens to have potent analgesic effects when it is given intra-muscularly. Toradol was never promoted as an oral medication because it was associated with an intolerably high incidence of gastro-intestinal bleeding. Still, it concerns me that it is often given to patients who may already be taking another NSAID medication. The use of two NSAIDs together potentially increases the risk of gastro-intestinal complications, including bleeding. It also increases the potential for kidney problems that may result from anti-inflammatory medications decreasing renal (kidney) blood flow. Thus it is probably best if Toradol is avoided or not used for any significant length of time in those patients already on non-steroidal anti-inflammatory medications.

Taking Pain Medicines Effectively

Now that I have familiarized you with the spectrum of choices of pain medications, I would like to address some other important considerations, which will help you understand how to take back control of your pain. Some patients will try to stretch out the interval between doses of medication out of fear of getting addicted to it. Unfortunately, in doing so, they allow the pain to break through to the point where they are intermittently incapacitated by it. Instead of feeling like you are on a roller-coaster ride with your pain, it may be preferable to put yourself on a regular schedule of taking pain medication. This may allow you to function maximally in spite of your arthritic problems. Of course, this needs to be done under the auspices of your doctor. Your physician should give you guidelines regarding the maximum amount of pain medicine that you are permitted to take in any twenty-four hour period of time. These instructions should be strictly adhered to. If this proves to be an insufficient dose to control your pain, then you need to make that clear on your next visit. The doctor then can increase the dose or change your pain medication to something stronger.

The timing of your pain medication is important. If you know that you are about to drive a motor vehicle, it is best if you do not take a narcotic medicine. These medications may have a sedating effect on you. You could then end up injuring yourself or others due to the side effects from your pain medication.

In Step 11, I will discuss the importance of the timing of your pain medicine prior to sexual activity. This will allow you to enjoy the pleasure of sex without the interference of your aches and pains. If you are gainfully employed and have a job where you need a clear head, then you may want to avoid any heavy dosages of painkillers prior to going to work. Obviously this needs to be balanced out with any musculo-skeletal pain, which could prevent you from performing the requirements of your job.

Many patients complain about pain that awakens them from their sleep. One of the nice things about the controversial drug, Oxycontin, is that it delivers a slow release of the pain medication that is able to control the pain throughout the night. This helps patients get a restful night's sleep. MS Contin, which is released in the body in a similar way, also can accomplish this. The Duragesic patch also is capable of delivering medication around the clock via the skin. Most other narcotic medicines are required to be taken every four to six hours. They then dissipate as they are metabolized in the body. One helpful tip is to place your "middle of the night dose" along with a glass of water on the nightstand so that you will be prepared if the pain awakens you during the night. This will prevent you from having to get up, while still half asleep, and somehow make your way to the bathroom. Once there, you then fumble around trying to find your pain pill. If you have everything already prepared at the bedside, it is much more likely that you will be able to quickly get back to sleep after taking your needed medication.

Some of my patients seem far more worried about getting addicted to their pain medications than they are about adequately controlling their pain. I feel that this is often a big mistake. Uncontrolled pain interferes with every aspect of your life. It may prevent you from being able to work. It may interfere with your marital situation and your sex life. It may cast a shadow over other activities that you used to enjoy. The pain may discourage you from participating in rehabilitation exercises and aquatics. This could be far more detrimental to your arthritis than your theoretical concerns about addiction to your pain medication.

Some patients may avoid taking narcotics because of problems with constipation. It is important that you start on a prophylactic program for constipation in anticipation of this problem. Don't wait until you are impacted or having to strain while on the commode before you take action. Be sure to take plenty of fluids including fruit juice. You should take a stool softener (which is a soap in a capsule) to make the stool easier to pass. You should increase the fiber in your diet and may wish to add Fibercon tablets, Metamucil, Benefiber, or an alternative powdered fiber mixed in water. Prunes or prune juice are good natural remedies. If you have used all of these things and are still getting constipated, then you may need to add Senekot-S once or twice a day. It does contain a laxative and, therefore, should not be used on a regular basis without your doctor's approval. Milk of Magnesia tablets or liquid is another way of "opening things up." Otherwise you might end up requiring an enema, and this is no picnic!

If you are truly going to take back control of your arthritis, then you are going to have to find ways to adequately control your pain, so that the pain does not dominate you and ruin your life. Your physician will be best able to advise you on which medication to take and at what dose. Don't undermine your doctor's instructions by incorrectly under-medicating yourself because of your own fears. If you have the opposite problem of having a doctor who is not responding to your complaints about your pain and reluctant to prescribe pain medication, then you may need to change physicians. Physicians will be anxious for you to eventually enroll in some type of physical rehabilitation program. This may enable you to improve to the point that your analgesic medications can be gradually withdrawn or eliminated. In the past, rheumatoid arthritis sufferers have often required narcotic pain medications in order to get through each day. The advent of biologic therapies, which I will discuss in Step 5, has so dramatically benefited many rheumatoid arthritis patients, that they no longer have the same need for pain medications. Pain medication, however, may be a necessary remedy during flares of your disease. It may allay your suffering so that you can carry on gainful employment in spite of significant arthritic involvement. Look to these medicines as being one important component of your overall treatment program.

Alternative Ways to Control Pain

There are numerous other ways to control pain in addition to using medications. Hypnosis, if done by a qualified hypnotherapist, can be very beneficial. Audiotapes can be made for you to assist you in incorporating self-hypnosis into your program. Techniques can be learned which will allow you to be able to block out the pain using your mind rather than drugs. In fact, self-hypnosis can duplicate the same sensation that you get after your pain medicine kicks in, without actually taking the pill.

Psychological and psychiatric consultation and treatment may also help some patients learn how to better cope with the pain. Anti-depressant medications can have a beneficial effect on your degree of pain and should be considered, even if you are not feeling particularly depressed. Nerve pain, such as occurs with neuropathies, may respond to Neurontin, Tegretol, or Zonegran more than it might to just mild narcotics.

Physical therapy may also be helpful in alleviating your pain. The use of modalities like ultrasound, electrical stimulation, massage therapy, and hot packs may be beneficial. This is especially true if you have a significant component of muscular spasm and pain. A transcutaneous nerve stimulator (TENS unit) placed on the skin can block pain in the back or in a limb. Acupuncture may be helpful and provide some individuals with temporary relief. It is often covered by insurance carriers when it is prescribed by a physician. It has not been shown to be of any lasting value in inflammatory forms of arthritis.

Sometimes when there is a persistent area of muscle tenderness (tender point or trigger point), an injection into the muscle of an anesthetic (numbing) medicine like xylocaine, either alone or in combination with cortisone can eliminate this muscle pain. An injection of the same combination of drugs into the epidural space of the spine (which is outside of the spinal cord itself) can alleviate sciatica (nerve pain radiating down the back of the leg). A series of epidural steroid injections may be given once a week for three weeks to control the more severe bilateral leg pains that are associated with spinal cord pressure from narrowing of the spinal canal (spinal stenosis) secondary to arthritis or severe disc disease. Some patients with persistent low back pain that has failed all other treatments may need to have a spinal cord stimulator implanted to control the pain.

If a patient has a significantly ruptured disc in the cervical or lumbar spine, which does not respond to medical treatment, then it may be most appropriate to consider surgery to alleviate the symptoms and remedy the situation. A neurosurgeon or orthopedic spinal surgeon should evaluate the patient and see if surgery would have a high chance of remedying the situation. In a patient who has completely lost the joint space in a particular joint, such as the hip or knee, then it may be necessary to consider joint replacement surgery and an orthopedic surgeon should be consulted. Thus, surgery offers an alternative solution to help in eliminating or improving your pain, if conservative medical management has failed to do so. Your rheumatologist will be able to discuss this with you to determine if you have exhausted every option short of having surgery. The rheumatologist will also be aware of whether you could be hurting yourself in any way by holding off on undergoing surgery sooner rather than later.

A New Electrical Device for Arthritis

For those patients suffering from osteoarthritis of the knee, a new device is now available that has been shown to decrease pain and possibly provide benefit to the remaining cartilage in the joint. The unit is called the BioniCare BIO-1000 and is worn over the knee joint at night while the patient is sleeping. The strength of the electrical impulse is lowered by the patient so that the individual is not aware of the stimulation being delivered to the joint. In one study patients noted decreased knee pain even after just one month of usage. Their function in the joint also improved. Sixty per cent of patients with severe osteoarthritis, who were candidates for joint replacement surgery, were able to postpone their surgery for up to four years with use of this device. A study is currently underway to assess efficacy for use over the hip joint. Patients desiring more information about this unique approach to controlling knee and hip pain secondary to osteoarthritis can go to www.bionicare.com on the Internet or call them at 1-800-BIO-KNEE.

Using Joint Injections to Treat Painful Joints

Patients who are experiencing arthritic pain that is localized to one or two joints may have their pain markedly diminished by the injection of cortisone directly into the joint. If a patient has widespread joint involvement as part of their inflammatory arthritis, then it may be more appropriate to treat the condition systemically with medication that will potentially improve all of the joints simultaneously. Even in the latter situation, however, if there is one joint that stands out as being worse than the others, then it still could be injected in addition to the systemic medication.

In painful osteoarthritis of the knee, instillation into the joint with a preparation of hyaluronic acid may alleviate the pain for many months. The most commonly used products are Synvisc, Hyalgan, and Supartz. These are given on a weekly basis for three weeks and must be injected directly into the joint. There is a very small chance of post-injection inflammation with swelling and pain, but if this occurs it is generally easily remedied. For the most part, however, these injections are well tolerated and beneficial.

In order to take back control of your arthritic and musculo-skeletal pain, you need to be familiar with all of these options that I have presented to you. Perhaps only one or two of them will be needed to control the pain in your particular case. In more complicated situations, you may need to try most of these in order to get enough relief to get through each day. You and your doctor, working together to try to combat your pain, will be able to work through all of these many choices and figure out what is best for you.

Key Points in Taking Back Control of Your Pain:

1. Make sure to communicate to your doctor the degree of pain you are experiencing.

2. Find a doctor who assesses your level of pain at each encounter.

3. Try different pain medications starting with the mildest first and then escalating up the ladder towards the strongest medicines until your pain is adequately controlled.

4. Be careful not to exceed the recommended dosages of pain medicines including acetaminophen (Tylenol).

5. Try to work out the timing of your doses so that you are not always waiting for the pain to become severe before you first think about taking your pain medication.

6. Don't take strong potentially sedating narcotics right before operating a motor vehicle.

7. Time the dosages of your pain medicine to enable you to function better at work or at home and even in anticipation of sexual activity with your significant other.

8. Prepare ahead of time for pain that may awaken you in the middle of the night by placing an extra tablet on the nightstand with a cup of water or switching to a longer acting medication.

9. Don't let your fear of addiction to pain medications blind you to the far greater benefits that you may get from taking adequate pain medication.

10. Be aware of alternative ways of controlling your pain, such as with physical therapy, massage, hypnosis, trigger point injections, a TENS unit, epidural steroid injections, intra-articular steroid injections, viscosupplementation, and surgery.

11. Do not allow your pain to become the dominant force in your life.

Step 4: Take Back Control of Your NSAIDs (Non-Steroidal Anti-Inflammatory Drugs)

Telltale Signs That You Need More Knowledge About NSAIDs:

- You are not certain as to whether you should be taking a traditional NSAID or one of the newer COX-2 selective NSAIDs.

- You are not sure whether you should simply be taking acetaminophen (Tylenol) versus being on an NSAID.

- You are currently taking Coumadin as a blood thinner and are wondering which NSAID you should take, if any.

- You have heard about some controversy regarding Celebrex and Vioxx and this has made you fearful of taking these.

- You have marginal kidney function and want to know if it is safe for you to take any of the NSAIDs.

- You have a history of a prior stomach ulcer and are concerned about the risk of a recurrence due to taking an NSAID.

- You are over age sixty-five and are unsure if there are special safety considerations for you.

- Due to the expense of your NSAID, you would prefer to cut down on your dosage or the frequency of dosing in order to save money, but you are not sure if this is the right thing to do.

Why NSAIDs Work

Most patients with arthritis will be treated at some point in time with an anti-inflammatory medication. Over thirty years ago researchers had discovered that substances called prostaglandins were found in inflamed and arthritic joints in excessive quantities. An enzyme called cyclo-oxygenase was critical in the generation of these inflammatory mediators. It was also discovered that aspirin taken in sufficient quantities was capable of blocking or inhibiting this cyclo-oxygenase enzyme, thereby decreasing the joint inflammation.

Subsequently other non-aspirin compounds were discovered which could also block this inflammatory pathway. Although cortisone (a corticosteroid) was also able to inhibit this enzyme, these new drugs were different from corticosteroid medicines. Thus, these medicines were named non-steroidal anti-inflammatory drugs (NSAIDs). Over the last three decades, multiple NSAIDs have been synthesized, all of which have been demonstrated to control arthritic inflammation. The list includes ibuprofen (Motrin), naproxen (Naprosyn), diclofenac (Voltaren), piroxicam (Feldene), indomethacin (Indocin), sulindac (Clinoril), and numerous others. In the last few years, the NSAID field has been complicated further by the introduction of a new group of anti-inflammatory medicines called selective COX-2 inhibitors, namely celecoxib (Celebrex), rofecoxib (Vioxx), and valdecoxib (Bextra).

In order for you to take back control of your arthritis, you will need to gain a better understanding of the benefits and risks of these NSAIDs. This knowledge will help prevent unnecessary complications that may occur in association with these medicines.

Table 4.1
The Newer Selective COX-2 Inhibitors

Brand Name	Generic Name
Celebrex	celcoxib
Vioxx	rofecoxib
Bextra	valdecoxib

Acetaminophen versus NSAIDs

First of all I need to address the issue of acetaminophen (Tylenol) versus NSAIDs in the treatment of osteoarthritis, the most common type of arthritis. The current treatment guidelines from the American College of Rheumatology indicate that patients with osteoarthritis should first be tried on acetaminophen before proceeding to an NSAID. In a minority of patients, acetaminophen used in amounts up to four grams per day may be sufficient to provide patients with adequate pain relief. NSAIDs, however, provide additional benefits including decreased stiffness, decreased swelling, and increased mobility. Thus, most patients with osteoarthritis do, in fact, end up moving on to an NSAID at some point.

Also many patients are surprised to learn that it's not necessarily an "either or" situation when it comes to NSAIDs and acetaminophen. As an analgesic (pain medicine), acetaminophen can be added to full doses of an NSAID medication as long as it is given in doses that don't exceed 4000 mg per each twenty-four hour period. Other stronger pain medicines can also be substituted for acetaminophen in conjunction with an NSAID, if the pain is not adequately controlled. It is true that NSAIDs themselves have pain-relieving qualities, but sometimes this effect is not sufficient to control all of the pain. The over-the-counter use of lower doses of NSAIDs such as ibuprofen, Aleve, or Orudis was in part designed to promote these medications for mild to moderate types of pain, headaches, or the discomfort from menstrual cramps, in addition to arthritis. Unfortunately, some folks do not understand that these still are NSAIDs with all of the potential associated risks. Some patients, who are already on another prescribed NSAID, will mistakenly supplement with one of these over-the-counter NSAIDs. This just increases the likelihood of incurring a serious side effect related to NSAIDs. Also it is important to note that patients should not be taking over-the-counter NSAIDs over a prolonged period of time without proper monitoring by a physician.

GI Issues with NSAIDs

The major problem with traditional NSAIDs is that they may lead to significant gastro-intestinal (GI) side effects including stomach ulcers, GI bleeding, perforations in the stomach or intestines, and blockage internally (obstructions). A number of ways to get around these potential side effects have been devised. Patients are instructed to take NSAIDs "sandwiched" in the middle of a meal to use the food to help "buffer" against any irritation of the stomach lining. If the patient has a prior history of GI problems or is experiencing symptoms, then the doctor may decide to simultaneously place you on what is termed a histamine receptor antagonist (e.g., Tagamet (cimetidine), Zantac (ranitidine), or Pepcid (famotidine)). An even more potent group of medications for these problems falls under the category of protein pump inhibitors (PPIs) and includes Prilosec (omeprazole), Nexium (esomeprazole), Prevacid (lansoprazole), Protonix (pantoprazole), and Aciphex (rabeprazole). There has been some controversy about using these preventive medicines in combination with NSAIDs due to the increased cost involved. There is also concern that these GI medications might mask symptoms until a patient presented with overt bleeding or a full-blown ulcer. It may be just as economical for a patient to purchase the more expensive COX-2 selective drugs with their safer gastro-intestinal profile, as it is to take a traditional NSAID along with one of these GI "meds" used to treat the stomach symptoms. If you are one of those lucky individuals with a cast-iron stomach, then you can probably get by on the less expensive, traditional

NSAIDs without developing any GI problems, but even in the "best" of stomachs the risk of these GI side effects always looms over you. "Hidden" blood loss can sometimes be picked up by noting the finding of anemia on a blood test. Thus a complete blood count (CBC) should be done at six-month intervals to make sure that this is not occurring. Any patient on NSAIDs who complains of black and tarry stools (melena) should be immediately evaluated for the possibility of gastro-intestinal bleeding. This could be secondary to the NSAID itself or due to some other underlying abnormality, possibly "brought out" by use of traditional NSAID treatment, which makes it easier for a gastro-intestinal lesion to bleed.

Issues About Kidney Function and NSAIDs

One area of concern that has not changed even with the advent of these new COX-2 selective drugs is the response of the kidneys to all of the NSAIDs—traditional and COX-2 selective inhibitors alike. All of these medicines potentially can decrease blood flow through the kidneys. This is true of Celebrex, Vioxx, and Bextra, as much as it is for the "old stand-bys" like Voltaren, Motrin, Naprosyn, and the rest of the group. In patients over sixty-five years of age, whose circulating blood volumes may be diminished and who also may have a degree of underlying kidney disease from other problems like hypertension or diabetes, there is particular risk of kidney complications from these medications. Every individual taking an NSAID should be monitored periodically regarding his or her kidney (renal) function. In people with any type of higher risk, I would recommend checking the kidney blood tests (blood urea nitrogen (BUN) and serum creatinine) within one to two months after starting on a new NSAID to make sure that the drug has not adversely impacted the kidneys. Thereafter, the kidney tests may be routinely evaluated approximately every six months. Patients, who have significant renal impairment, are not good candidates to take NSAIDs at all, as these medicines could possibly throw them quickly into complete renal failure. If you are taking an NSAID, it is an excellent idea to keep yourself well hydrated. Dehydration combined with NSAIDs can be detrimental to your kidneys. So make sure that you drink six to eight glasses of fluid each day to help protect your kidneys.

COX-1 vs. COX-2 Inhibitors

Since I have been distinguishing between the newer selective COX-2 inhibitors and the older traditional NSAIDs regarding GI and renal side effects, now might be a good time to explain the differences between these medicines in more detail. In the 1990's, it was discovered that there are actually two distinct forms of an enzyme (called cyclo-oxygenase) that are involved in the synthesis of a substance called prostaglandin. There are some parts of the body where these prostaglandins are necessary for normal physiologic functions. This type of cyclo-oxygenase enzyme is called COX-1 and is termed a "constitutive" (physiologically necessary) enzyme. When inflammation from arthritis occurs in a joint, prostaglandins are generated by a different cyclo-oxygenase enzyme. The particular cyclo-oxygenase enzyme that is "turned on" under these circumstances is called COX-2 and is considered an "inducible" form of the enzyme, as it is only brought on or "induced" with inflammation. Once it became apparent that there was a more specific enzyme involved with the arthritic process itself, an intense research effort was begun to find a way to specifically block this enzyme without blocking the COX-1 needed for the body's ordinary biologic functions. The first selective COX-2 inhibitor to be developed was Celebrex. This has been followed by the subsequent release of the COX-2 inhibitors Vioxx and Bextra.

Since only COX-1 is found in platelets, the COX-2 selective drugs do not interact with platelets. Platelets are circulating cells in the body involved in the formation of clots. Traditional NSAIDs including aspirin can inhibit the clumping together of platelets, which can be beneficial in the prevention of heart attacks or strokes. It can, however, potentially be detrimental if there is GI bleeding and the platelets are inhibited from forming clots to help stop the bleeding. One of the reasons that there are fewer cases of GI complications, including bleeding, with the newer selective COX-2 inhibitors may be related to this lack of interference with the body's platelets.

Unlike aspirin and other traditional NSAIDs, the fact that COX-2 selective NSAIDs do not promote bleeding makes them particularly advantageous in patients who are on "blood thinners" (anti-coagulants) like Coumadin for other medical problems. One of the major side effects of Coumadin is internal bleeding, and therefore, physicians are reluctant to prescribe traditional NSAIDs in combination with Coumadin. COX-2 selective drugs like Celebrex, Vioxx, and Bextra are safer choices to be used in this setting. It is still advisable to monitor prothrombin blood tests ("protimes" and INR's) when COX-2 inhibitors are prescribed in a patient already on Coumadin therapy.

Although I have pointed out some of the unique safety features of the newer COX-2 specific NSAIDs, it is important to understand that their efficacy is similar to the traditional NSAIDs if both are taken in the correct amounts. The older NSAIDs inhibit both the COX-1 and the COX-2 enzymes, so that the enzyme involved with joint inflammation is indeed blocked with these medications. The problem is that at the same time, they are also blocking the COX-1 enzyme inadvertently, and this creates a number of the side effects that we would prefer to avoid when treating patients. The new COX-2 inhibitors, therefore, are not some kind of "super aspirins" or "wonder drugs," but rather just a much more targeted type of treatment for arthritis that is safer, but not more efficacious than older types of NSAIDs.

Taking NSAIDs Correctly

There is one important principle that I would like you to understand and appreciate when you are trying to take back control of your NSAIDs and your arthritis. If you are taking an NSAID to treat your condition, you must take it in the fully prescribed dose on a regular basis. If you repetitively miss or skip doses, then you may not achieve an anti-inflammatory level of the medicine in the bloodstream and will not maintain that level on a long-term basis. If you only take the drug sporadically, you may be experiencing some pain relief due to its analgesic effect, but you will not be getting the much needed anti-inflammatory effect required to suppress your rheumatic disease. Patients will often cut down on their NSAID dose on their own due to the expense of the pills, side effects, or just a lack of motivation to stick to the program. It is particularly difficult to remember to take medicines on a three or four times a day schedule. Once-a-day drugs have the highest rate of compliance. Paradoxically, in the elderly patient it is safer to prescribe medicines in divided doses. The once-a-day medications have a longer half-life, which means that they are metabolized more slowly. In the older patient, there is the potential for these once-a-day drugs to accumulate in the body and therefore, lead to potential side effects. So on the one hand, once-a-day medicines are easier to remember to take, but on the other hand they may be more dangerous in older patients with a decreased rate of metabolism.

Clearly not everyone has to be switched over to the newer COX-2 selective inhibitors, especially if they are doing well on their traditional NSAID. Many patients are able to tolerate these older NSAIDs without any significant side effects. This still, of course, doesn't absolutely guarantee that that same patient couldn't suddenly experience a GI bleed, but this is less likely to occur in an otherwise healthy individual. Patients, who have had a prior history of ulcer disease or bleeding, are considered high-risk patients when it comes to NSAIDs. These folks are definitely candidates for the newer, safer NSAIDs.

Controversy Surrounds COX-2 Inhibitors

As you are reading this discussion of the benefits of the newer NSAIDs from a safety standpoint, I am sure that some of you are wondering what the fuss on television and in the newspapers was all about concerning Vioxx and Celebrex. Actually the problem had to do with a Vioxx research study, but Celebrex got dragged into the fray due to "guilt by association," since it was also a COX-2 selective drug. This controversy stemmed from a rheumatoid arthritis study on Vioxx at a 50 mg per day dosage compared with Naprosyn. Unfortunately, in their zeal to enroll patients, some doctors entered a number of rheumatoid arthritis patients who also had serious cardiac problems. One of the drawbacks for these particular individuals was that the design of the study did not permit them to take their once-a-day aspirin while participating in this trial. As might be anticipated, a number of patients developed heart attacks, and the number on Vioxx exceeded those on Naprosyn by a four to one ratio. This is not totally unexpected due to the anti-platelet effects (similar to aspirin) seen with Naprosyn. Vioxx, on the other hand, does not interact with platelets. Researchers have analyzed the data to try to explain the increased incidence of heart attacks in the Vioxx group. No one has yet convincingly demonstrated that Vioxx actually promotes the formation of blood clots. Instead, what has been shown is that Vioxx and the other COX-2 selective drugs do not block platelet function. Thus, a patient who has a higher risk of a future heart attack or stroke should probably be taking one coated aspirin tablet daily in conjunction with Vioxx, Celebrex, or Bextra. By doing this, patients do give up some of the GI safety benefits of taking COX-2 inhibitors without aspirin, but the combination is still safer than taking a traditional NSAID.

NSAIDs and the Liver

There are other potential side effects with NSAIDs that need to be considered. Liver toxicity has turned out to be a relatively minor concern in healthy individuals. Clinoril (sulindac) may be associated with a 2% incidence of a form of hepatitis that reverses once the drug is stopped. Voltaren (diclofenac) and other NSAIDs may cause liver function test abnormalities in 2% or fewer patients. Therefore, it is necessary to include periodic monitoring of liver tests along with the other laboratory studies that I have mentioned. NSAIDs would not normally be recommended in patients with active hepatitis infections. This is the case in acute infectious hepatitis A, but also is particularly something to avoid with the increasing number of patients developing hepatitis B and C infections. If the hepatitis is quiescent with normal liver tests, then the risk of using NSAIDs in this setting is much diminished. If the virus is active and the liver function tests are markedly abnormal, then NSAIDs should be avoided. Remember that the liver is a major route of metabolism for the NSAIDs and if it is not functioning properly, then the drug could accumulate to potentially dangerously high levels in the body leading to other side effects.

As you can now appreciate, there are a number of major considerations in determining whether an individual affected with arthritis should be treated with an NSAID. Once the decision has been made to start therapy with an NSAID, then a physician needs to decide which NSAID to choose for that particular patient and at what dosage. It is also imperative that the treating physician knows exactly how to best monitor the patient to make certain that there are no major adverse consequences from these medicines. Of particular importance is ensuring that there are no problems with side effects in the gastro-intestinal organs, kidneys, or liver. A rheumatologist has special training in deciding which of the NSAIDs is right for you and your specific condition, and how to best monitor you to make sure that it is safe for you to continue on NSAID therapy.

Key Points in Taking Back Control of Your NSAIDs:

1. An NSAID may help you by not only decreasing your pain, but also by increasing your mobility and decreasing your stiffness.

2. Be careful when taking the over-the-counter forms of NSAIDs. Do not add these to another physician-prescribed NSAID. Do not take these in high doses on a long-term basis without being monitored by a doctor.

3. While on an NSAID make sure that you are being monitored regularly for any GI side effects, as well as kidney or liver problems.

4. If you are considered a high-risk patient for GI problems, then you are a candidate for the newer COX-2 selective NSAIDs.

5. If you are considered "at-risk" for a heart attack or stroke, you may need to take a one-a-day aspirin along with the newer COX-2 selective NSAIDs.

6. The COX-2 selective NSAIDs are safer to use in patients who are also taking blood thinners (anti-coagulants).

7. The new COX-2 selective inhibitors are superior in safety, but are considered equal in efficacy to the traditional NSAIDs.

8. NSAIDs are best avoided in patients with significant kidney disease or active liver disease.

9. Patients over sixty-five years of age should be monitored more closely when on NSAIDs. Keep yourself well hydrated while taking this type of medication. Go in for regular check-ups with your doctor.

10. In order for NSAIDs to truly help you, they need to be taken at the prescribed dosage and on a regular basis. If you only take your NSAID on a sporadic basis, you may get some pain relief, but you will not get the anti-inflammatory benefits that will help control your arthritis.

Step 5: Take Back Control of Your Disease-Modifying Anti-Rheumatic Drugs (DMARDs) and Biologic Response Modifiers (BRMs)

Telltale Signs That You May Be a Candidate for DMARDs or BRMs:

- You have inflammatory arthritis, for example rheumatoid arthritis or psoriatic arthritis, but it is not being controlled by the use of NSAIDs combined with pain medication.

- You have been told that your x-rays show evidence of erosions of the bones at your joints, and that this may portend the development of future deformities and disability.

- You are on corticosteroid therapy and have been unable to taper the dose down without a flare-up of your disease.

- The pain from your arthritis is causing you to rely more on stronger pain medications in order to control your symptoms.

Why You Need to Take Control of Your DMARDs and BRMs

There are over one hundred types of rheumatic conditions, and they range from mild musculo-skeletal disorders to very severe and aggressive forms of inflammatory arthritis. The mildest forms of joint and muscle pain may be readily managed with NSAIDs or simple analgesics for pain relief. In more significant forms of inflammatory arthritis, such as rheumatoid arthritis, this type of treatment is inadequate to control the severe inflammation taking place in the synovial lining of the joints (synovitis). Stronger treatments directed at the immune system are required to quiet down this inflammatory response or even potentially to control it completely, i.e., induce a remission of the arthritis. For the last fifty years, rheumatologists have selected from an ever-expanding menu of disease modifying anti-rheumatic drugs (DMARDs) that can interfere with this inflammation. In the last few years much more targeted treatments directed at those proteins specifically involved in causing the joint inflammation and damage have been developed. These treatments called biologic therapies or biologic response modifiers (BRMs) are capable of controlling inflammatory arthritis to a much greater extent. Unlike the DMARDs, these BRMs have shown a propensity to not only arrest the joint inflammation, but also to block or even (in some cases) reverse the damage (as seen on x-rays) in the joints.

As a patient suffering from arthritis, you should totally educate yourself about these revolutionary treatments. Once you have done this you will be able to have some input into the various treatment options available to you. You should press your doctors to at least discuss and possibly consider these therapies in your particular case. A physician, who is not a rheumatologist, may be much less familiar with the benefits of the new biologic treatments and may, therefore, be less inclined to strongly recommend them. Consequently, you may need to be proactive as far as a referral to a knowledgeable rheumatologist, who can initiate these treatments if indicated. These therapies have a much higher likelihood of putting your disease into remission and preventing you from developing significant deformities and disability. It is, therefore, critical for you to be knowledgeable about these therapies. A board-certified rheumatologist should be able to decide if your situation is indeed one that would be responsive to DMARDs and/or BRMs.

Understanding DMARDs

Disease-modifying anti-rheumatic drugs (DMARDs) are a group of medications that can modify the symptoms and joint changes associated with a rheumatic condition. Anti-inflammatory medications (NSAIDs) are designed to deal with the day to day swelling, inflammation, and stiffness in the joints, but are not felt to have significant long-term benefits. DMARDs on the other hand appear to interact with the immune system in the body to help control the basic disease process. They usually work in a slower more prolonged fashion and thus sometimes are also called slow-acting anti-rheumatic drugs (SAARDS). Also occasionally you will see these medicines referred to as "second line agents" with the first line of therapy being the nonsteroidal anti-inflammatory drugs or mild pain medications. The DMARDs are then added to the "mix" when NSAIDs alone are inadequate in controlling the patient's symptoms. Recent research studies, however, have made it clear that earlier utilization of DMARDs results in a better long-term outcome for patients. Since these medicines have a slower onset of action than NSAIDs or corticosteroids (e.g., prednisone), starting them earlier in the disease course allows them to "kick in" more quickly and prevent further damage to the joints.

Table 5.1
Disease-Modifying Anti-Rheumatic Drugs (DMARDs)

Medication Name
Plaquenil (hydroxy-chloroquine)
Azulfidine (sulfasalazine)
Gold therapy
D-penicillamine
Methotrexate
Imuran (azathioprine)
Arava (leflunomide)
Sandimmune (cyclosporine)
Prograf (tacrolimus)

A Malaria Treatment (Plaquenil) That Can Benefit Rheumatic Disease Patients

At a time when interest in "natural" remedies is running high, it is only appropriate to focus on a DMARD, which actually was discovered in the early 1800s in the bark of the Cinchona tree in Peru. Chloroquine and the hydroxylated form of Chloroquine called Plaquenil (hydroxychloroquine) are actually used to treat malaria, but they have been found to also be effective in rheumatic diseases like rheumatoid arthritis and systemic lupus erythematosus (SLE). Plaquenil is the most commonly used anti-malarial drug for rheumatic disorders and is felt to interact with the immune system in numerous ways to accomplish its disease modifying benefits.

I mentioned that anti-malarials might play a role in the treatment of systemic lupus erythematosus. This is especially true in patients with photosensitivity or with lupus skin lesions. Anti-malarials are able to counteract the negative effects of ultraviolet (UV) light. UV light can have a detrimental effect in systemic lupus erythematosus by stimulating the formation of the anti-DNA antibodies involved in disease flare-ups. Plaquenil can rapidly work to improve lupus skin lesions and can have sustained effect even long after the Plaquenil has been discontinued. Subsequent recurrent skin lesions can be re-treated with Plaquenil therapy.

Plaquenil not only works for skin involvement in SLE, but also is effective in controlling the joint symptoms associated with active lupus. Thus, anti-malarial medication not only serves to improve symptoms, but also has the ability to decrease the requirement for corticosteroids (e.g., prednisone). It is, therefore, considered "steroid-sparing." Since we are always concerned about the long-term effects of high-dose steroids (e.g., osteoporosis, cataracts, weight gain, diabetes, hypertension), any medication that enables the patient to reduce or eliminate the use of corticosteroids is considered beneficial.

Plaquenil is an example of one of our DMARD therapies, but I mentioned previously that another term for this group of medications is SAARDS or slow acting anti-rheumatic drugs. In fact, Plaquenil may take months to begin to exert its positive effects. Although it is considered one of the milder DMARDs, it has shown benefit in anywhere from 50 to 75% of patients using it. It is also one of the least toxic and best tolerated of all of the DMARDs.

The side effect that receives the most attention with Plaquenil has to do with potential damage to the eyes. Plaquenil may be associated with changes in the macular portion of the retina leading to visual impairment. This is, however, an extremely rare finding if the dose of Plaquenil does not exceed 400 mg per day. Rheumatologists are aware of this fact and normally prescribe only 200 mg once or twice daily. There is an ongoing debate on how often your eyes should be examined when you are taking Plaquenil. Rheumatologists have been trained to order an eye exam every six months, whereas, many ophthalmologists feel that annual examinations are sufficient. Personally, I always prefer to be safe rather than sorry, and so I am in the "every six-month camp." If the ophthalmologist finds changes in the retina, then the Plaquenil should be discontinued to avoid any progressive and more severe changes in the eyes.

Other potential side effects of Plaquenil include gastro-intestinal symptoms such as nausea or vomiting, but these are not common. A violet colored skin rash may occur in the extremities (called a lichen planus eruption). Less commonly, patients may develop central nervous system side effects including seizures. As I stated above, in the vast majority of patients none of these problems occur and Plaquenil is extremely well tolerated. This clearly differentiates it from the other DMARDs where the incidence of side effects can be quite troubling.

Plaquenil can be utilized as a single DMARD (monotherapy) in milder cases of rheumatoid arthritis. It also has been shown to be helpful as one part of a combination treatment with multiple DMARDs. Plaquenil has even been used as part of a "triple-therapy" cocktail in conjunction with Azulfidine (sulfasalazine) and methotrexate. In these studies, the use of all three drugs together was superior to utilizing methotrexate by itself, or Plaquenil combined with just the Azulfidine. Other studies have shown added benefits of prescribing Plaquenil simultaneously with methotrexate. Researchers have noted that Plaquenil may actually protect the liver and cut down on liver function abnormalities that may be seen with methotrexate alone. Plaquenil, therefore, can be an extremely helpful drug in combatting rheumatic disease. It is especially advantageous because of its excellent safety profile. In patients with more severe and aggressive forms of rheumatoid arthritis, however, it is usually too weak of a DMARD to completely control the disease process.

Azulfidine (sulfasalazine): A Drug That Works for the Wrong Reason

Often, anti-rheumatic therapies turn out to work for reasons different from the original rationale involved in their development. This certainly was true in the creation of a drug called Azulfidine (sulfasalazine or SSZ), which combines an antibacterial treatment called sulfapyridine with an anti-inflammatory drug called salicylic acid (aspirin). The original incorrect premise was that rheumatoid arthritis was an infectious condition that should lend itself to antibiotic treatment. It turns out instead that the drug is effective due to its beneficial effects on the immune system and not as an antibiotic.

Where does SSZ fit into our treatment paradigm? It appears to be more effective than Plaquenil, which I have indicated is more appropriate as a single therapy only in very mild disease. One study comparing Plaquenil and SSZ showed fewer erosions with SSZ over a three-year period. It appears, however, to be somewhat less efficacious than methotrexate, although this varies in different studies. European rheumatologists have used SSZ a great deal in the treatment of another form of inflammatory arthritis called ankylosing spondylitis. American rheumatologists started prescribing it more frequently approximately twenty years ago. It has also been effective for the treatment of psoriatic arthritis. The usual dosage is anywhere from two to three grams per day, if tolerated. Unfortunately, gastrointestinal side effects can be a dose-limiting factor with this drug. Similar to most of the other DMARDs, the percentage of patients who can tolerate SSZ on a longer-term basis drops off to only 20% after five years of treatment.

Patients on SSZ may experience side effects including gastrointestinal symptoms of nausea, vomiting, loss of appetite, abdominal pain or indigestion. Some patients may develop dizziness or headaches. Less than 5% of patients may note a rash. Certainly this medication would not be recommended for patients with a strong history of sulfa allergy. Patients need to be monitored regarding any decreases in the white or red blood cells as well as for the development of liver function abnormalities. There have been reports of interference with male fertility. Therefore, SSZ would need to be discontinued in male patients who desire children.

Whatever Happened to Gold and D-penicillamine Therapy?

At the end of the nineteenth century gold compounds were prescribed for the first time for the treatment of tuberculosis. In the early 1900s, scientists reasoned, albeit incorrectly, that rheumatoid arthritis may be caused by similar microbacterial organisms. Gold treatment was, therefore, used in this condition as well.

Gold was administered principally by intramuscular injection. It was in common use until the 1980s when it was replaced as the most frequently prescribed DMARD by methotrexate. An oral form of gold (Auranofin) that was a fairly weak DMARD never really gained significant status among disease modifying treatments.

It was largely due to problems with toxicity, the lack of long-term benefits, and the advent of newer and better treatments that led to a decline in the use of gold therapy. Prior to these newer medications, gold was being utilized in both adult and juvenile forms of rheumatoid arthritis, psoriatic arthritis, as well as ankylosing spondylitis. Although gold salts were shown to have various beneficial effects on biologic functions in the body, it was not totally clear how it worked in rheumatoid arthritis. It was certainly a typical SAARD with a three to six month period of time before one would start seeing its positive effects. In clinical studies, the benefits from gold therapy lasted an average of just over two years. One out of four patients demonstrated some x-ray improvement in the joints in some studies. When compared with methotrexate, gold measured up fairly well in efficacy, but there was a marked reduction in the incidence of side effects with methotrexate compared with gold. Similar to what happened with other DMARDs, the vast majority of patients gradually discontinued their gold treatments due to these side effects or lack of efficacy. Only one out of five patients still remained on gold therapy after five years of treatment.

Side effects with gold treatment were intolerably high and occurred in approximately one out of every three patients. These included skin rash and mouth or tongue irritation and ulcerations. More troubling was the development of gold-induced kidney disease with protein and red blood cells found in the urine. Gold therapy also had the potential to severely lower a person's platelet count. On rare occasions, this even led to fatal consequences. Other blood cells were sometimes affected due to bone marrow suppression from the gold. Once rheumatologists became comfortable with the once weekly dosage of methotrexate without encountering some of the disturbing toxicity seen with gold injections, then gold treatment ended up being consigned principally to chapters on the history of DMARDs and no longer serving as an important treatment option.

A similar fate awaited another DMARD called D-penicillamine (Depen), which had its brief period of enthusiastic support until an awareness of its toxicities led to its demise. D-penicillamine is a "cousin" to the antibiotic penicillin. Although there are a number of theories, it was never totally clear how D-penicillamine worked in rheumatoid arthritis. Clinical studies showed that D-penicillamine seemed to be similar in efficacy to other DMARDs like gold, Plaquenil, and Imuran (azathioprine).

Toxic side effects that led to its decline in usage included severe reductions in the various blood cells in the body. It also caused significant kidney disease with protein in the urine. A worrisome neurologic condition called myasthenia gravis characterized by muscle weakness occurred in some patients treated with D-penicillamine. Other autoimmune problems included drug-induced lupus and polymyositis or dermatomyositis. Even though rheumatologists tried to reduce the dosage originally recommended to avoid these side effects, it still became increasingly difficult to be able to administer this particular DMARD without running into significant problems. In the end, rheumatologists abandoned this potentially toxic treatment and moved on to methotrexate and newer therapies.

Methotrexate: The Most Commonly Used DMARD

Dermatologists had been using methotrexate for years to treat cutaneous forms of psoriasis long before rheumatologists finally adopted the once-a-week dosaging for use in rheumatoid arthritis.

Methotrexate has now been in use as a treatment of inflammatory arthritis since the late 1980s.

There has been some debate about whether methotrexate works primarily as an anti-inflammatory drug or as an immunosuppressive drug. Clearly, when patients are treated with methotrexate, some individuals develop significant infections as a consequence of therapy. This would imply that the patient's immune system certainly has been influenced by the methotrexate. This is particularly true of the higher doses of methotrexate that are used to treat cancer, rather than the low doses typically utilized in rheumatoid arthritis. Methotrexate does lead to increased levels of a substance called adenosine, which has anti-inflammatory properties. Methotrexate also appears to influence proteins (cytokines) involved in inflammation. The anti-inflammatory effects from methotrexate could explain why it seems to work within a matter of weeks, compared with other slower acting medications that take months to exert their immunosuppressive effects.

Early on, there was some concern about the use of methotrexate in combination with NSAIDs, but this turned out not to be a significant worry when using the low doses of methotrexate prescribed in rheumatoid arthritis. This could potentially be more of an issue in patients receiving methotrexate as chemotherapy in higher doses. Methotrexate levels are not influenced by taking it with food. Some patients may experience gastrointestinal upset with oral methotrexate, but it is acceptable to take this with a meal to counteract those side effects. One interaction that may be important involves patients with gout who are taking benemid (Probenecid). This treatment for gout may interfere with the kidney's ability to excrete methotrexate and could result in increased drug levels of methotrexate. Thus, this combination of medications should be avoided.

Clinical research studies have shown that the benefits from methotrexate may become obvious within three to four weeks of starting the drug. If patients then subsequently discontinue their methotrexate, a flare could be expected as soon as three to four weeks afterwards. Comparison studies with other DMARDs have generally shown superior results with methotrexate. When methotrexate was compared to Imuran (azathioprine) for example, it was superior with fewer side effects. After nearly one year of treatment, far more patients were able to tolerate the methotrexate versus those continuing with the Imuran. In some clinical studies, methotrexate also was equivalent in its benefits to injectable gold, but with far fewer side effects. Methotrexate was also shown to be superior to another immunosuppressive drug called cyclosporine. With methotrexate, patients have been able to subsequently reduce their NSAIDs as well as their corticosteroids as their symptoms improved. Methotrexate has shown the ability to decrease the erythrocyte sedimentation rate (ESR) along with joint pain and swelling. The average length of time that patients are able to continue treatment with methotrexate is twice that of the other disease modifying anti-rheumatic drugs. Thus, not only is methotrexate highly beneficial, but due to its excellent safety profile, patients tend to continue with weekly methotrexate for more prolonged periods than other DMARDs.

One drawback of methotrexate is that many patients treated with this medicine are considered only "incomplete" responders. These patients have partial rather than complete remissions. Methotrexate has not been found to be as effective as biologic response modifiers in terms of preventing erosions, although it may slow the rate of destruction.

Combination treatment of methotrexate along with one or more DMARDs has often led to an increased number of side effects without marked additional improvement in outcome. This has certainly been true when methotrexate has been combined with gold or combined with Imuran (azathioprine). The combination of methotrexate with sulfasalazine or cyclosporine, however, may offer some additional potential benefits. Methotrexate when combined with Arava (leflunomide) may help "partial responders" on methotrexate, but this is at the risk of incurring increased liver toxicity with the two drugs together.

For over the last ten years, methotrexate has been considered "the backbone" of therapy for rheumatoid arthritis patients. With the advent of biologic response modifiers (BRMs), the best "combination" treatment has been the use of weekly methotrexate together with one of the new biologic agents. Methotrexate is also an important therapy in the treatment of psoriatic arthritis resulting in decreased activity in the psoriatic skin lesions along with improvement in joint pain and swelling. Methotrexate has been used for other rheumatic conditions, including polymyalgia rheumatica and temporal arteritis with patients who have had difficulty getting off of prednisone without flare-ups. Methotrexate has also been successfully utilized in systemic lupus erythematosus, polymyositis or dermatomyositis, as well as adult onset Still's disease and juvenile rheumatoid arthritis.

When given on a daily basis, methotrexate turns out to be far too toxic. Once-a-week doses, however, are able to prevent some of these undesirable side effects. Methotrexate can be given in tablet form or as a liquid that can be mixed with juice. It can also be given by injection in the muscle, particularly in those patients who have experienced gastrointestinal problems (nausea, vomiting or diarrhea) with the oral form of methotrexate. Intra-muscular injections are also recommended for those patients who need to be given higher doses, which are not normally well-tolerated orally. The maximum dose that can usually be given by mouth is 20 mg per week. The intramuscular route allows the patient to receive doses ranging as high as 25 to 50 mg per week.

Normally patients are prescribed folic acid tablets (1 mg daily) to help prevent some of the toxic side effects with methotrexate. This particularly helps prevent irritation or ulceration over the tongue or inside of the mouth. Studies have shown that giving the folic acid does not diminish the efficacy of the methotrexate. Folinic acid (leucovorin) also works to decrease side effects, but it is more expensive than the over-the-counter folic acid and requires a prescription. If folic acid is not doing the job, however, then folinic acid would be a good second choice.

One of the most worrisome potential toxicities with methotrexate has to do with liver function abnormalities. Years ago, patients with long-term methotrexate had to undergo regular liver biopsies to make certain that there were no pathologic changes. These studies, however, showed that although there might be mild changes present, there was no significant cirrhosis (permanent scarring). Patients with hepatitis B or hepatitis C infection or with a history of alcohol-related problems would not be considered good candidates for methotrexate. Patients are actually warned not to drink alcohol while undergoing treatment with methotrexate.

Some individuals will note extreme fatigue after taking their methotrexate, and this may occur particularly within the immediate first twenty-four hours after their dose. One alternative is to try to spread the dosage over three twelve-hour time periods to give less of a dose at one time. Otherwise, these patients may only be able to tolerate extremely low doses of methotrexate.

One unusual problem with methotrexate is the development of multiple nodules (nodulosis) most commonly over the hands or feet. Rheumatoid arthritis itself can be associated with nodule formation, but one would ordinarily expect that a treatment designed to control rheumatoid arthritis would decrease the presence of nodules, not aggravate them. In some patients, lowering the dose may help, while others have had some benefit with concomitant use of Plaquenil, Azulfidine, cyclosporine, colchicine, or even prednisone. If the nodules multiply or increase in size, then methotrexate may need to be discontinued.

If you are already on methotrexate or are considering this drug, one of the most important things you can do is make certain you are under the care of a physician who has had a great deal of experience using methotrexate and knows how to properly monitor you. Methotrexate can affect the blood cells in the body, and therefore, your blood count needs to be checked on a monthly basis. Worsening kidney function can lead to increased levels of methotrexate in the body which, in turn, could lead to other toxicities. Dosage reductions, therefore, would be necessary in the face of kidney disease. Liver tests (by blood studies) need to be obtained monthly as well. Significant changes in your liver enzymes could necessitate a reduction in the methotrexate dose or discontinuing it altogether.

Rarely, methotrexate can cause a potentially life threatening condition in the lungs called "methotrexate lung." Due to this risk, some doctors recommend getting a baseline chest x-ray before starting treatment with methotrexate. Certainly if any significant symptoms of shortness of breath or chest pain occur while a patient is on methotrexate, a chest x-ray should be obtained to make sure the patient is not experiencing this complication. If present, "methotrexate lung" needs to be treated aggressively with folinic acid, cessation of the methotrexate, and possibly high-dose corticosteroid therapy.

Female patients, who decide that they want to try to get pregnant after being on methotrexate, need to wait approximately six months before conceiving. Methotrexate can interfere with the formation of a normal, healthy fetus and it would be prudent to stay off of this drug for a six-month period to avoid any risk of congenital abnormalities in one's offspring. Male patients wanting to start a family should wait a minimum of three months before attempting to conceive.

As mentioned previously, methotrexate is sometimes associated with serious infections including more unusual types of infections. Patients who develop fever and other localized symptoms of infection should be evaluated as quickly as possible and started on appropriate treatment. Once a diagnosis has been made, methotrexate should certainly be withheld while an infection is being treated so as to not further exacerbate its severity.

This leads us to the issue of whether methotrexate should be withheld in patients who are about to undergo surgery. Certainly this appears to be a prudent thing to do so as to cut down on the risk of any post-operative infectious complications. Surgeons are also concerned about any potential interference with wound healing or with increasing the risk of wound infection. There have been studies, however, which have shown the ability to continue methotrexate in spite of surgery without always having dire consequences. In my own practice, however, I generally withhold the methotrexate for at least one week prior to surgery and only restart the methotrexate when the wound is satisfactorily healed.

Thus, methotrexate has been the "king of DMARDs" since its approval in 1988 for the treatment of rheumatoid arthritis. I have tried to point out a number of caveats that you should be aware of if you are thinking about going on methotrexate or already taking this drug. It should be obvious to you that since there are so many "nuances" with the administration of methotrexate therapy, that you are best served by being in the hands of someone highly experienced in its use. This will result in a much lower incidence of adverse events and will allow you to remain on this drug for a more prolonged period of time.

Arava (leflunomide): An Alternative to Methotrexate Therapy

Similar to methotrexate, a DMARD called Arava (leflunomide) works in patients with rheumatoid arthritis by interacting with the immune system. Previous research studies have shown that Arava seems to work as effectively as methotrexate. The studies have also suggested some prevention of the progression of x-ray findings in the joints. Side effects have included diarrhea, hair loss, skin rash and liver toxicity. The diarrhea generally can be controlled by decreasing the daily dosage or by using anti-diarrheal medications such as Imodium or Lomotil. The hair loss also can be diminished by decreasing the dose of Arava. If it is more severe, then the hair loss may only resolve if Arava is discontinued. Patients need to be watched closely regarding liver function abnormalities. This requires similar monitoring to that performed with methotrexate patients. Less than 5% of patients will have more worrisome types of elevations of the liver tests.

Recently, Public Citizen and its director, Dr. Sidney Wolfe filed a petition asking the FDA to pull Arava off the market based on twelve patients who died from liver failure. These included patients who were being properly monitored by their physicians, but who died precipitously in spite of this. In the petition, Dr. Wolfe also voiced his concerns about high blood pressure as well as a potentially fatal allergic skin reaction (called Stevens-Johnson syndrome).

It is absolutely imperative that female patients taking Arava use birth control while on this drug. There is considerable worry about the potential for congenital abnormalities. Most doctors would recommend terminating any pregnancy that develops while a woman is on Arava. In a female desiring to conceive, it is recommended that she be off this drug for a minimum of two years before doing so.

Patients also need to be monitored regarding their blood counts including the platelet cells, which are needed for proper clotting in the body.

Arava has been studied in combination with methotrexate and the combination did lead to improvement in half of the patients. There was a trade-off, however, with an increased frequency of liver function test abnormalities along with diarrhea and hair loss in patients on the combined medicines. In the studies that have been done, Arava has shown comparable efficacy to methotrexate and sulfasalazine.

Arava is given orally, most often with a three-day loading dose of 100 mg per day followed by a maintenance dosage of 20 mg daily. As noted above, in patients experiencing side effects with diarrhea or hair loss, the daily dose can be reduced to 10 mg daily. If the side effects continue, then the Arava would need to be discontinued.

Arava, therefore, offers an alternative treatment to those patients who are not completely controlled on methotrexate or who have experienced side effects with methotrexate that necessitated discontinuation of this drug. Patients need to be monitored on a regular basis by a physician experienced with this DMARD. Proper monitoring would certainly help to cut down on any potential toxicity. There still may be some risk, however, as pointed out by Dr. Wolfe, even when Arava is given by the most knowledgeable physician. Certainly, the risks of toxicity from Arava need to be balanced against the potential benefits that a patient might derive.

Reversing the "Pyramid" Approach to the Treatment of Rheumatoid Arthritis

For many years rheumatologists were trained to treat rheumatoid arthritis by starting off with the least toxic medications first and only advancing to stronger treatments if patients failed to respond to the simplest modes of therapy. This required observing and monitoring patients for at least a six-month period before instituting more aggressive forms of treatment.

Nowadays, this concept of slowly ascending a treatment "pyramid" towards the strongest and potentially most toxic medications at the top of the pyramid has been abandoned. Clinical studies have now shown that if a physician waits to start aggressive treatment for months in a patient with erosive rheumatoid arthritis, valuable time is lost. Patients with x-ray abnormalities have a high likelihood of deteriorating further with the subsequent development of deformities and associated disability. Thus, rheumatologists now treat patients very aggressively and are unwilling to wait for the patient to experience advanced disease before instituting these potentially beneficial and stronger medications. In a patient with active rheumatoid arthritis with multiple swollen and tender joints, rheumatologists would certainly consider starting methotrexate. Then if the patient did not completely respond or had x-ray evidence of bony erosions at the joints, methotrexate might be combined with one of the new tumor necrosis factor inhibitors. In patients who failed to respond to Enbrel, Humira, or Remicade, then Kineret, another biologic response modifier (an Interleukin-1 inhibitor) could be recommended.

Clearly, if there is greater than a six-month delay in a primary care physician referring an active rheumatoid arthritis patient to a rheumatologist to receive these new therapies, then this could put the patient at risk for the subsequent development of deformities and disability. Patients who are trying to take back control of their arthritis should be aware of this. A patient should insist on seeing a knowledgeable board-certified rheumatologist who can help make the right decisions on appropriate DMARD therapy as well as the concurrent use of biologic response modifiers. Don't let yourself be "bamboozled" by a physician, who does not have sufficient expertise, telling you that this type of evaluation or specialized treatment is not necessary. Try to find the most knowledgeable doctor in your area to help you figure out the best treatment program for your condition.

Use of the Prosorba Column in Rheumatoid Arthritis

In those patients who have failed to respond to multiple DMARDs or who cannot tolerate them due to side effects, another option is passing their blood through a specially designed column. This is called a Prosorba protein A immunoabsorption column, a medical device approved for the treatment of rheumatoid arthritis. It is not completely clear how this treatment works. With this procedure, the patient's whole blood is passed through a cell separator so that the plasma is divided from the red blood cells. The plasma is then passed through a column, which contains a substance called protein A (derived from staphylococcus organisms). As a result of these treatments, a sub-group of rheumatoid arthritis patients will improve. The treatment does not appear to permanently affect the patient's immune system in any way as is the case with a number of the DMARDs.

Patients usually receive one treatment weekly for twelve weeks with these treatments each lasting two hours at a time. In prior studies, approximately 42% of individuals had a 20% improvement in their joint pain and swelling with benefit lasting anywhere from six weeks to over one year.

If patients did not respond to the initial twelve-week course of treatment, they did not tend to benefit from subsequent treatments. Patients who feel better with the initial treatment may improve with a second course of treatment. There are some side effects associated with this treatment including gastrointestinal symptoms with nausea, vomiting, diarrhea and abdominal pain, as well as fatigue, chills, fever or flushing. There is also a small incidence of low blood pressure.

Patients, who are on angiotensin converting enzyme inhibitors (ACE inhibitors) for hypertension, should be off of these for at least three days before undergoing a Prosorba treatment. This treatment is not recommended in patients with known clotting disorders. It should be used cautiously in patients who have a history of abnormal kidney function or low blood pressure. It also could present a potential problem for patients with known congestive heart failure whose symptoms might be aggravated with the shifting of fluid in and out of the body. The Prosorba column also might pose a problem for patients who are significantly anemic.

Thus, the use of this Prosorba column in patients who have failed many DMARDs presents an alternative treatment to control the acute symptoms of rheumatoid arthritis. It is not a commonly performed procedure and not all insurance plans cover it. Certainly with the advent of biologic agents, it has been largely put on the back burner as a significant treatment option in rheumatoid arthritis.

Is There Any DMARD Treatment for Fibromyalgia?

Disease modifying anti-rheumatic drugs are supposed to change the course of the underlying condition. The physician's and patient's greatest expectation would be a complete remission with cessation of any active symptoms. The treatment of fibromyalgia syndrome includes a complex regimen designed to deal with a patient's chronic pain, muscle spasm, tender points, and frequently associated fatigue. The groups of medicines utilized to improve patient's symptoms may include muscle relaxants, antidepressants, sleep medications, pain medicines (analgesics), and NSAIDs. The combination of these drugs may certainly lead to less muscular pain, more restful sleep, and even less fatigue. None of these medicines, however, is able to truly modify the long-term course of fibromyalgia or induce a significant remission. Thus, when it comes to treating fibromyalgia syndrome, we do not really refer to any of these drugs as DMARDs. Instead, these are symptomatic treatments that certainly may work to make the fibromyalgia patients condition better, but are not expected to arrest it altogether.

Are There Any DMARDs for the Treatment of Osteoarthritis?

In osteoarthritis there is a problem with degenerative changes taking place in the cartilage that covers the ends of bones that meet within a joint. The chondrocyte is the cell present in the cartilage responsible for synthesizing the correct "building blocks" to make healthy cartilage. In osteoarthritis, for whatever reason, these cartilage components become defective. This leads to cartilage that more readily deteriorates. Research continues in an effort to try to pinpoint whether there are genetic factors leading up to this faulty synthesis of cartilage versus some underlying immunologic problem. The treatment of osteoarthritis involves the use of NSAIDs, pain medications, injections of cortisone or viscosupplements into the joint, and surgery. There is no data yet to support the use of medications that suppress the immune system when it comes to dealing with osteoarthritis. There is research taking place, however, to see if biologic therapies may have a future role in the treatment of osteoarthritis.

Glucosamine and chondroitin sulfate have become extremely popular supplements used by osteoarthritis patients. A study done in Belgium in 1999 showed a decrease in knee pain in osteoarthritis patients who were treated with glucosamine versus those treated with only a placebo pill. The investigators also concluded that in their study glucosamine resulted in preservation of the cartilage or even improvement in cartilage thickness. Critics of this study rightfully felt that plain knee x-rays were an inaccurate way of assessing knee cartilage and that special views of the knees or even MRI (magnetic resonance imaging) studies were required in order to truly show any long-term benefit in the cartilage. A more sophisticated study is currently being undertaken by the National Institutes of Health (NIH) here in the United States. Clearly if cartilage thickness could be shown to increase with this treatment, then we would have to think of glucosamine and chondroitin therapy as disease modifying. As of this writing, however, there is no true DMARD proven for the treatment of osteoarthritis. As our knowledge of the underlying causes of osteoarthritis become more apparent, perhaps investigators will discover novel ways of truly "modifying" outcomes in osteoarthritis, rather than merely providing patients symptomatic relief.

Tumor Necrosis Factor (TNF) and Its Role in Inflammatory Arthritis

Tumor necrosis factor is one of the most critical proteins (cytokines) involved in the inflammatory process in the joints of patients with inflammatory arthritis (e.g., rheumatoid arthritis, psoriatic arthritis, and ankylosing spondylitis). It is produced by cells called macrophages involved in the body's defenses, as well as the lining cells of joints (synoviocytes). In rheumatoid arthritis patients, researchers have found increased levels of TNF in the joints as well as in the serum.

Tumor necrosis factor may be detrimental in a number of ways. It stimulates a substance that allows white blood cells to move outside of the blood vessels. They then move into the joints where they then may participate in the inflammation and damage that subsequently takes place. TNF increases the production of a substance called metalloproteinase, which is damaging to the joints. Tumor necrosis factor also stimulates the production of another one of the protein (cytokine) culprits in arthritis called interleukin-1. Thus, it is easy to understand why it is important to find ways to block the detrimental effects of tumor necrosis factor. This is why pharmaceutical corporations have focused on tumor necrosis factor inhibitors and have synthesized these revolutionary biologic response modifiers.

Table 5.2
Currently Approved Biologic Response Modifiers (BRMs)

Medication Name	Usual Dosage	Route of Administration
Enbrel (etanercept)	50 mg weekly	sub-cutaneous injections
Remicade (infliximab)	3 to 10 mg/kg every two months	intravenous infusions
Humira (adalimumab)	40 mg every two weeks	sub-cutaneous injections
Kineret (anakinra)	100 mg daily	sub-cutaneous injections

Enbrel (etanercept) Leads the Way As the First Approved Biologic Response Modifier

The development of Enbrel as a biologic response modifier is one of the most exciting developments in rheumatology in the last fifty years. Investigators were successfully able to synthesize what is termed a fusion protein, which was capable of inhibiting tumor necrosis factor. This protein essentially acted in a sponge-like manner to soak up the TNF in the body as it was being released.

The original studies showed that Enbrel worked best by administering 25 mg by subcutaneous injections twice a week. Since it was made from human components, the rheumatoid arthritis patients did not form antibodies to the Enbrel. Fifty-nine per cent of patients had at least a 20% improvement in their joint pain and swelling after six months of treatment. Fifteen per cent of patients achieved a 70% rate of improvement after six months of therapy.

More recent data has indicated that 50 mg of Enbrel given once-a-week works as well as 25 mg twice-a-week. In time, patients will, therefore, be switched over to this once-a-week regimen.

Enbrel does cause problems in slightly over one third of patients with injection site reactions. These tend to be mild to moderate in severity and tend to occur in the first few weeks of treatment. With further injections, these eventually resolve.

There is always a concern when prescribing TNF inhibitors about the potential for increasing the risk of infection. We instruct our patients to hold off on their Enbrel injections with the onset of any signs of a possible infection and to contact the doctor for immediate evaluation and to assess the need to initiate antibiotic therapy.

Although there is some controversy about this, there is no hard evidence to suggest an increased risk of malignancy with the use of Enbrel treatment. There have been cases of activation of dormant forms of tuberculosis, although this has been even more of a problem with Remicade. Patients should have a PPD skin test prior to starting Enbrel. If this is positive, then treatment with Isoniazid (INH) for nine months needs to be instituted. Enbrel is not recommended in patients with multiple sclerosis (MS) because of concerns about this form of biologic therapy aggravating demyelinating neurologic disorders like MS. Patients should have periodic blood counts drawn to make sure that these are not being adversely affected by the Enbrel.

There has been such a strong demand for Enbrel that Immunex (now owned by Amgen) had trouble keeping up with production requirements. During the spring of 2002, there were some serious shortages. These have now been remedied by the opening of new factories. As with some of the earlier DMARDs, the decision as to whether to start Enbrel and whether to use it as a single agent or in combination with a DMARD such as methotrexate is best left in the hands of a knowledgeable rheumatologist who makes these decisions on a regular basis.

Table 5.3

Side Effects with Biologic Response Modifiers

Name of Medication	Cytokine it Inhibits	Side Effects
Enbrel (etanercept)	tumor necrosis factor (TNF)	Injection site reactions, activation of TB, infections, worsening of multiple sclerosis, problems with severe heart failure patients
Remicade (infliximab)	tumor necrosis factor (TNF)	infusion reactions (with hives, shortness of breath, low blood pressure), activation of TB, infections, worsening of multiple sclerosis or heart failure, positive anti-nuclear antibodies or lupus-like symptoms
Humira (adalimumab)	tumor necrosis factor (TNF)	injection site reactions, infections, activation of TB, worsening of multiple sclerosis or heart failure
Kineret (anakinra)	Interleukin-1 (IL-1)	injection site reactions, infections

Remicade (infliximab): The First Intravenous Biologic Therapy

Following the approval and release of Enbrel, a second tumor necrosis factor inhibitor called Remicade (infliximab) was approved. This had previously shown to be of benefit in a type of inflammatory bowel disease called Crohn's disease. Studies, however, showed that it also was highly effective in the treatment of rheumatoid arthritis. Unlike Enbrel, which is a fusion protein, Remicade is actually an antibody towards tumor necrosis factor (TNF). Remicade combines mouse and human components in this antibody. After a series of "loading" type doses over a six-week period, maintenance Remicade therapy is then usually given every eight weeks. Occasionally some patients require higher doses of Remicade and even may need it more frequently on a monthly basis.

Originally, there was concern about patients forming antibodies towards the mouse portion of the Remicade molecule. When Remicade was first being utilized, it was recommended that methotrexate be used concurrently to help control and suppress this antibody formation. It now appears that it is not absolutely necessary to do this and that Remicade, in fact, can be used as monotherapy (single therapy) without concurrent methotrexate.

Normally, patients are started on a Remicade dosage of 3 mg per kilogram of body weight (1 kg equals 2.2 lbs). If the patient, however, does not appear to be responding to a series of infusions at this dose, then this can gradually be increased upwards to a maximum of 10 mg per kilogram.

Nursing personnel are trained to handle any reactions that may take place during the approximately two-hour Remicade infusion. There is some evidence that patients, who have been on Remicade for long periods of time without any prior complications, may actually be given the infusion over a shorter period of time. Originally patients receiving these infusions have complained of side effects including headache, nausea, dizziness, skin rash including hives, or lowered blood pressure. At six months time, over half the patients achieved a 20% improvement in their joint symptoms.

Patients starting on Remicade need to have a PPD skin test prior to commencing treatment. If the skin test for tuberculosis is positive, then similar to Enbrel patients, they will need to be treated for a nine-month period of time with Isoniazed (INH). As with Enbrel, there are similar concerns with Remicade regarding the risk of infection and avoiding this treatment in patients with multiple sclerosis. Patients need to be monitored not only regarding their blood counts, but also for the development of any positive antinuclear antibody (ANA) and DNA antibody results. A positive ANA would not be an automatic reason to stop the Remicade as long as the patient did not develop typical symptoms of a drug-induced lupus syndrome. Drug-induced lupus may manifest itself by a skin rash, pleurisy, joint and muscle aching, low-grade fever, hair loss, or ulcerations in the nose, mouth, or vagina.

Patients with shortness of breath and ankle swelling who are diagnosed with severe congestive heart failure (CHF) are not considered good candidates for Remicade treatment. Originally it was hoped that TNF inhibitors might be beneficial in this group of patients, but in fact, the opposite scenario has panned out and Enbrel, Remicade, and Humira are now to be avoided in this setting.

Remicade may have negative impact on patients with demyelinating disorders like multiple sclerosis. In patients who are suspected of having one of these neurologic conditions, it is best not to utilize Remicade therapy.

With the advent of these biologic agents, there has always been a theoretical concern about whether manipulating the immune system could result in an increased incidence of malignancy. Although this has been reviewed by the FDA, there has not been any concrete evidence yet to support this worry. Patients with rheumatoid arthritis are already at a higher risk of developing lymphomas. It is difficult, therefore, to ascribe the new onset of lymphoma in a rheumatoid arthritis patient to a biologic agent, when it may have occurred secondary to the rheumatoid arthritis itself.

Remicade has not only led to improvement in patients' joint pain and swelling, but also in decreased damage found on x-rays of the joints. Remicade can have a dramatic impact on the course of rheumatoid arthritis and the response can be fairly swift following the first few Remicade infusions. Not only have patients noted rather dramatic resolution of their symptoms, but many patients have been able to reduce a number of their other medications, including their corticosteroids, their NSAIDs, as well as eliminating other DMARDs. Not only does this result in a cost savings to the patient, but it reduces the potential toxicities associated with these other medications and this is certainly beneficial to the patient.

Humira (adalimumab): Yet a Third TNF Inhibitor

In December of 2002, the FDA approved another biologic treatment called Humira (adalimumab). Like Enbrel and Remicade before it, this biologic response modifier blocks tumor necrosis factor (TNF). Both Enbrel and Humira are self-administered by injection just under the surface of the skin (sub-cutaneous injections). This differs from Remicade, which is given by intravenous infusion. Like Remicade, Humira is actually a monoclonal antibody against TNF.

The recommended Humira dosage is 40 mg given every two weeks. Since not too many people are fond of getting stuck with a needle on a regular basis, the every two weeks regimen is somewhat more convenient and less odious than the once or twice weekly Enbrel shots. Another advantage of Humira is that it is composed of entirely human components. This differentiates it from Remicade, which consists of a combination of mouse and human elements. Some Remicade patients experience reactions to the mouse portion of the Remicade molecule. Humira (being a totally humanized monoclonal antibody) does not elicit any such antibodies against it. That being said, like Enbrel, Humira patients may experience injection site reactions. These tend to be mild and usually resolve after the first few weeks of treatment.

These reactions may be alleviated by applications of ice, or treatment with antihistamines or steroid cream. Rotating the sites of injection over the anterior abdominal wall and thighs may help to avoid skin reactions.

Some of the same concerns that I expressed with Enbrel and Remicade still need to be raised with Humira. Patients who are candidates for Humira treatment need to be screened with a TB skin test. If this is positive, then they need to be properly treated in order to avoid activation and dissemination of previously dormant tuberculosis organisms. Also anyone with a history of significant recurrent infections would be at risk with any of the TNF inhibitors including Humira. This biologic agent should be withheld following the onset of a significant infection with prompt evaluation and treatment by a physician.

Humira also poses a risk for patients with a history of significant congestive heart failure. It should be avoided in patients with multiple sclerosis or similar types of neurologic disorders. Similar to Enbrel and Remicade, there is no hard evidence to prove that Humira increases a patient's chances of developing cancer. An association with lupus-like symptoms is extraordinarily rare with Humira, although some patients may certainly convert to a positive antinuclear antibody test (ANA).

Besides all of these side effect issues, patients are also confronted with the problems of the high cost of these treatments and issues of insurance coverage. Enbrel and Humira both are currently priced at approximately $13,500 per year. The lowest dose of Remicade at 3 mg/kg is in the same ballpark. If the number of vials of Remicade given intravenously doubles or triples in order to more adequately control a patient's inflammatory arthritis, then the price goes up accordingly. Medicare does cover the cost of intravenous therapy, but without a supplemental insurance plan, this would still leave 20% of the expense uncovered. For many individuals, this makes Remicade unaffordable. Medicare currently does not pay for subcutaneous injections, which eliminates any possibility of reimbursement for Enbrel and Remicade. When Humira was launched, Abbott Pharmaceuticals decided to offer Humira free of charge to those Medicare patients who did not have drug prescription benefits. Their strategy presumably was to offer this service in the hope that Congress would eventually pass a Medicare prescription drug bill, as they did. This new legislation should help patients with the expense of these biologic therapies.

Humira has shown the ability to significantly improve patients' swollen and tender joints in studies that have lasted up to three years in duration. Sixty-four per cent of patients had a 20% improvement in their joint assessments (ACR-20), while approximately one quarter of participating patients had a 70% improvement (ACR-70). Patients also noted significant improvement in their functional capacity. Humira also was able to prevent the radiologic (x-ray) progression of rheumatoid arthritis. All of these benefits combined to prevent erosive and destructive disease in the joints. These beneficial effects are known to result in a decreased percentage of patients who develop deformity and subsequent disability. Clearly all three of these TNF inhibitors represent a major advance in the treatment of inflammatory arthritis.

Another Culprit in Inflammatory Arthritis Called Interleukin-1 (IL-1)

Besides tumor necrosis factor (TNF), a second culprit in the perpetuation of the joint inflammation seen in rheumatoid arthritis and other forms of inflammatory arthritis is called interleukin-1 (IL-1). This is a protein (cytokine) that allows communication between cells. Interleukin-1 is particularly detrimental to cartilage as well as bone. Tumor necrosis factor and Interleukin-1 interact with one another. Inhibiting TNF does partially block Interleukin-1, but not completely. Interleukin-1 is able to contribute to the destruction of cartilage and bone by stimulating the production of substances called matrix metalloproteinases, which are damaging to these tissues.

It is unfortunate that researchers have not been able to identify an initial cause or "spark" that sets off rheumatoid arthritis. If we knew this, perhaps we would be better able to prevent it from even starting up in an individual patient. What we do know is that once the disease begins, proteins (cytokines) are synthesized which stimulate further inflammation to develop. Thus, even though there is a certain level of frustration with our inability to truly prevent rheumatoid arthritis, rheumatologists are now extremely excited about biologic response modifiers that are able to block these protein signals.

Over many years, we have observed that some patients with rheumatoid arthritis may experience low-grade fevers, especially during the first year of disease activity. Other patients complain of weight loss or of a decrease in the size of their muscles. It turns out that these cytokines (TNF and IL-1) may be contributing to some of these symptoms seen in association with rheumatoid arthritis.

Although I have indicated that tumor necrosis factor and Interleukin-1 are important factors involved in the inflammation and destruction seen in rheumatoid arthritis, there are differences between them. TNF is mainly involved with the inflammation seen in rheumatoid arthritis, whereas, Interleukin-1 has greater impact on the bones and cartilage.

Normally, the body is able to combat the presence of damaging proteins like TNF and IL-1 with natural inhibitors. In rheumatoid arthritis patients, however, there is an imbalance in favor of these damaging proteins (cytokines). This outstrips the ability of the body's natural inhibitors to neutralize these proteins.

For example, the body makes a natural inhibitor of Interleukin-1, called IL-1Ra (Interleukin-1 receptor antagonist), which in normal situations can block the destructive effects of Interleukin-1. In rheumatoid arthritis, however, too much Interleukin-1 is present and this overwhelms the natural inhibitors that the body makes. In order to block Interleukin-1 successfully, a synthetic Interleukin-1 receptor antagonist had to be synthesized, and this was finally accomplished with the development and approval of Kineret (anakinra), which is now available to patients.

Kineret (anakinra): A BRM Against Interleukin-1

Kineret (anakinra) is a biologic response modifier that targets and inhibits Interleukin-1 in the treatment of rheumatoid arthritis. In order for this to work effectively, it has to be administered on a daily basis by self-injection under the skin at 100 mg per day.

It is currently indicated in patients who have failed at least one previous DMARD. It may be kept in reserve for those patients who have failed to respond to either Enbrel or Remicade, or simply utilized in a situation where patients have only gotten a partial or inadequate response from methotrexate treatment.

There has been some concern about the risk of infection with the combination of a TNF inhibitor with an Interleukin-1 inhibitor like Kineret. Studies are ongoing to obtain more data on this issue. For the time being, this combination is not being recommended. Kineret as a biologic agent, however, can certainly be used in combination with other DMARDs, such as methotrexate.

The major problem that patients have experienced with Kineret has been the formation of injection site reactions. As with Enbrel injections, these reactions also usually occur within the first month of treatment and tend to be fairly mild. These can be treated with topical therapy including ice packs, steroid cream, or Benadryl cream to alleviate some of the symptoms.

Patients using alcohol to cleanse the skin prior to their injection should allow the alcohol to dry prior to self-injecting in order to avoid the burning sensation from the alcohol. Patients have learned to rotate their skin sites to avoid irritating one particular area with repeated injections.

Key Points in Taking Back Control of Your DMARDs and BRMs:

1. Familiarize yourself with the various DMARDs and BRMs currently available to treat arthritis.

2. Plaquenil is a useful DMARD in mild forms of rheumatoid arthritis as well as in systemic lupus erythematosus.

3. Azulfidine is a stronger DMARD that often compares favorably to methotrexate.

4. As a result of toxic side effects and a lack of long-term efficacy, use of injectable gold to treat arthritis has fallen out of favor.

5. Methotrexate is the most commonly prescribed DMARD in the U.S. and offers superior efficacy than other DMARDs with a better safety profile.

6. Arava is yet another DMARD analogous to methotrexate. This medication may be associated with potential liver problems as well as diarrhea and hair loss.

7. The prior more gradual approach to the treatment of inflammatory arthritis has been supplanted by a much more aggressive, more rapid institution of newer therapies to prevent deformity and disability.

8. Tumor necrosis factor (TNF) and Interleukin-1 (IL-1) are two of the main culprits involved in the inflammation and damage seen in the joints in inflammatory arthritis.

9. Enbrel and Humira are TNF inhibitors that are administered sub-cutaneously, and may result in transient injection site reactions.

10. Remicade is a TNF inhibitor given by periodic intravenous infusions.

11. TNF inhibitors should be avoided in patients with a history of chronic infections, severe congestive heart failure, or multiple sclerosis.

12. Patients who are candidates for the TNF inhibitors need to be screened for prior tuberculosis exposure, and if necessary, treated with Isoniazid (INH) in order to receive these biologic therapies without the added risk of developing tuberculosis.

13. Kineret, an Interleukin-1 inhibitor, is also given by sub-cutaneous injection and may produce mild injection site reactions.

14. Biologic response modifiers may be used as monotherapy or may be combined with DMARDs such as methotrexate.

15. Biologic response modifiers have revolutionized the treatment of inflammatory arthritis. You should consult a knowledgeable rheumatologist to determine if you are a candidate for any of these new forms of therapy.

Step 6: Take Back Control of Your Medication Costs Including Over-the-Counter Drugs

Telltale Signs That Your Medication Expenses Are Spiraling Out of Control:

- You often have to choose between paying for your medications versus buying food for yourself and your family.

- In order to afford your medication, you take it only every other day or every third day to try to make it last longer.

- Without telling your doctor, you stop taking your most expensive medications because you simply cannot afford them.

- Instead of taking your prescription medication from your doctor, you start delving into over-the-counter pills recommended to you by a friend.

- You are confused about whether you should be taking less expensive generic brands of your medications or should stick with the more "pricey" brand names.

Beware the Infomercial

One way that a number of you are throwing money out the window is with products sold to you via infomercials. These carefully orchestrated thirty-minute programs are designed to beguile you and sucker you into purchasing pills, creams, supplements, devices or any other product that can be effectively hawked to you in this format. In the medical infomercials, an individual sometimes dressed in a white coat and looking highly professional in stature makes a persuasive case for the item being sold. Then, the infomercial goes through a series of "sound bytes" that are testimonials for this product. During these testimonials, the following phrases are often uttered by enthusiastic users of the product. "This is the best I have ever felt." "I now have more energy than I have ever had." "My sex life has never been better." "I feel so much younger." "I can do so much more." "My fatigue is completely gone." "I have no more pain."

The infomercial may switch back once again to the professional person we saw at the beginning of the program to repeat the same message that we heard earlier on. Once again, this is frequently followed by more testimonials or a repetition of some of the previous ones. Apparently this pattern of alternating the "pseudo-scientific" information with claims from people who have presumably tried the product is an effective format. During the final portion of the program you are presented with "The Offer" which normally includes discounts if you "order now." Sometimes a second product and even a third product may be offered free in conjunction with a purchase of the first product. Frequently, the offers are "guaranteed" including a "money-back guarantee." They also are often cleverly packaged with a name that suggests some new special formula.

You need to be aware that a carefully designed infomercial is one of the shrewdest ways to separate you from your money. These infomercials have been tested on individuals to ensure their persuasiveness. The format is one that has been confirmed to work effectively. I have actually had an opportunity to speak to an individual who produces infomercials and came away with the feeling that almost any specific tablet, cream or product could be effectively sold to the public through a properly produced program. This is "Madison Avenue" at its very best and you should be fully aware of how powerful and persuasive these infomercials are. They appeal to your desire to have your pain and fatigue reduced. They hit directly at your need to have more energy and feel younger. It does not particularly matter to those who are selling you these products whether they have any hard scientific evidence (with double-blinded clinical research studies) to prove that these items are effective. Since these products are not regulated in any way by the government, the entrepreneurs behind these products are free to use these very persuasive thirty-minute production pieces to induce you to buy. This is their goal and they are highly successful at it. One way you can prevent yourself from falling victim to these infomercials is by writing down all of the information and checking with your doctor before you buy. Your doctor will be able to tell you whether the product involved has any merit whatsoever. In all likelihood, the answer in the vast majority of cases will be to "save your money" because there is no evidence of any benefit from that particular product.

Saving on Your NSAIDs

One of the most significant monthly expenses for many patients with arthritis is the cost of their nonsteroidal anti-inflammatory drugs (NSAIDs). This cost can vary from less than $20 per month to upwards of $160 per month depending on the individual's needs and choices. Generic forms of NSAIDs are, of course, a lot cheaper than the brand names. All of the newer NSAIDs released in recent years are not yet available in generic form. The traditional NSAIDs, which have been around for many years, now can be purchased in the less expensive generic versions. There is no real strong data to support the concept that generic forms of NSAIDs are less effective than brand name NSAIDs, although some patients may insist that the brand name versions work better.

One important piece of advice is to check with your insurance carrier and see which specific NSAIDs they cover. If your physician writes a prescription for a medicine that is not on this list, your co-pay could be significantly higher or it may not be reimbursable at all. It may be helpful for you to bring a list of the "recommended" medications with you to your physician visit so that your doctor is aware of your specific medication coverage.

Some of my patients are reluctant to change from one NSAID to another even though their insurance carrier is asking that they do so. You should realize that these "choices" by your insurance carrier usually don't have anything to do with specific efficacy or side effect issues. These commonly have to do with contractual arrangements between your insurance company and the pharmaceutical manufacturers. Basically your insurance carrier makes a greater profit on certain medications due to these hidden agreements. They will, therefore, put pressure on your physician to change you to a "covered medication" to hold down expenses and increase their profitability. It may not always be in your own best interest to change your therapy, but it seems that financial considerations usually win out in this situation.

Those patients who have a "strong" stomach lining without any history of any gastrointestinal (GI) problems have the most options as far as cutting their NSAID cost. Patients of mine who have "iron stomachs" are able to tolerate even high doses of aspirin without any gastrointestinal bleeding or ulceration. Using high-dose aspirin as your anti-inflammatory medication does pose a potentially greater GI risk than even traditional nonsteroidal anti-inflammatory drugs. The traditional drugs, in turn, pose a greater risk than the newer selective COX-2 inhibitors, such as Celebrex, Vioxx and Bextra. Those patients with a history of a prior gastric ulcer or GI bleeding will require the safest and most expensive approach when it comes to anti-inflammatory drugs and the treatment of their arthritis. These patients are considered at "high risk" and constitute the main group of individuals who should be targeted for the use of selective COX-2 inhibitors. If these patients are prescribed traditional NSAIDs, then they may need additional preventative gastrointestinal medications in order to avoid recurrent GI complications.

Thus, if you are fortunate enough to be one of those individuals without a history of any gastrointestinal problems

and you do not have any prescription insurance coverage, then
you may try to get by with enteric coated aspirin or Ascriptin
(aspirin plus Maalox). To get an anti-inflammatory effect from
aspirin, most patients have to take anywhere from twelve to
sixteen aspirin per day in divided dosages. It is possible to tell if
you are be ingesting too much aspirin by the development of
ringing in the ears (tinnitus). If this occurs, then it can be alleviated
by simply reducing the dose gradually until the ringing resolves.
Also your physician can confirm any evidence of aspirin toxicity
by simply measuring an aspirin (salicylate) level in your blood.

Another very inexpensive way to go when it comes to NSAIDs
is to take the over-the-counter forms of ibuprofen (Advil, Nuprin,
Mediprin or Motrin). These usually are available as 200 mg tablets.
In order to control arthritic inflammation, you would have to take
three or four of these tablets at a time up to four times a day with
food. Aleve is also available over the counter. This is similar to a
prescription drug called Anaprox, but in a reduced strength of 220
mg per tablet. In order to control inflammation with Aleve, you
may need two tablets twice or three times a day with food. There is
also another over-the-counter tablet Orudis KT 12.5 mg. You might
need to take anywhere from three to six tablets twice a day with
meals in order to get an anti-inflammatory affect. It is critically
important to understand that when you take these over-the-counter
medicines in the higher doses that are required to control
inflammation, you still need to be monitored for gastrointestinal
bleeding or any abnormal effects on your kidney function. Thus,
you still need to be under a doctor's care and supervised with
laboratory monitoring approximately every six months.

If your doctor decides that you need a prescription NSAID,
the expense will vary depending on whether or not you have
insurance coverage. Patients who subsequently develop
gastrointestinal side effects from these medications will incur
additional costs if they need to be treated with medications to

heal any irritation of the GI tract. This expense is of course superimposed onto the cost of the prescription NSAIDs. There are two groups of gastrointestinal medications in particular that are useful in this situation. The first group consists of the histamine (H_2) receptor antagonists. There are less expensive over-the-counter versions of these, including Tagamet, Zantac or Pepcid. This group of medications is not as efficacious as another group called the proton pump inhibitors (PPIs). One of these called Prilosec is now available in a generic form and this has dropped its cost considerably. The other medications in this group that are still available as brand name only include Prevacid, Nexium, Aciphex and Protonix. Certainly, the expense of combining a prescription NSAID with the cost of a prescription proton pump inhibitor would in most cases exceed the cost of just taking a selective COX-2 inhibitor by itself (e.g., Celebrex, Vioxx, or Bextra).

If you are a patient, therefore, who has had gastrointestinal problems with the prescription NSAIDs, it would still be reasonable to be switched over to one of the selective COX-2 inhibitor drugs (if you can tolerate them without needing additional expensive gastrointestinal medication). When one considers cost, it is necessary to include other expenses beyond that of just the medication itself. Patients with gastric ulcers and bleeding often are hospitalized and this usually is an extremely expensive proposition. If you have to miss work due to gastrointestinal side effects from these medications, then this also needs to be factored in as part of the cost analysis. Normally, a single daily tablet of Celebrex 200 mg, Vioxx 25 mg or Bextra 10 mg will run you approximately $70 to $80 per month. If you have to double up on any of these medicines and take them twice a day, then these medications will get even more expensive to take.

If you are being treated for osteoarthritis and subsequently start doing considerably better, you may actually be able to taper off of your NSAID. For example, if you have osteoarthritis limited to your knees and then receive Synvisc intra-articular injections with resolution of your pain, you may be able to get by without NSAID medications. Acetaminophen (Tylenol) offers patients a minimal risk of any gastrointestinal problems and certainly is a lot less expensive than prescription NSAIDs. It is important to understand that there is no evidence that taking nonsteroidal anti-inflammatory medications on a long-term basis blocks the progression of osteoarthritis in any significant way. Since you are not interfering with the disease process itself, you should be taking these medications and varying your dosage based on the presence and degree of symptoms you are experiencing. In rheumatoid arthritis, if there is an excellent response to biologic response modifiers such as Remicade, Enbrel or Humira, patients may actually be able to get off their NSAIDs completely or reduce their dosage. This will not only decrease the risk of gastrointestinal side effects and potential problems with kidney function, but will cut out one significant medication-related expense.

It is, therefore, important to understand these various treatment options depending on one's age, medical condition, degree of joint inflammation, severity of the pain and gastrointestinal history. Clearly those patients who are at the benign end of the risk spectrum can try to get by with much less expensive anti-inflammatory drugs. Patients at the severe end of the risk spectrum may be candidates for the newer selective COX-2 inhibitors. This is certainly something that you need to review with your physician to see if cost savings are possible without putting your health in jeopardy.

Saving on Your Methotrexate

Methotrexate (MTX) is the most commonly used disease modifying anti-rheumatic drug (DMARD). Most patients with rheumatoid arthritis will start out on a MTX dose of 7.5 mg to 15 mg once a week and then be advanced up to a maximum oral dose of 20 mg. In 1988 when methotrexate was approved, we only had the availability of 2.5 mg tablets. Patients, therefore, would be started out on three of these 2.5 mg tablets on a weekly basis. In the last several years, methotrexate has become available in larger sized tablets called Trexall. These come in 5 mg, 7.5 mg, 10 mg and 15 mg strengths. You need to check with your pharmacy regarding the relative costs of the generic methotrexate tablets versus Trexall. In some pharmacies, the generic tablets are cheaper, whereas in others the Trexall actually turns out to be less expensive. Also, you should check with your insurance carrier to see which form of methotrexate is a better deal for you. There is still another way to save an even more significant amount of money on the cost of your methotrexate. There is a liquid form of MTX that comes in a vial and was originally formulated to be injected into patients. One solution to the high cost of methotrexate is to learn how to use this liquid form of methotrexate and take it orally instead of by injection. This certainly requires careful instructions from your physician and training from his or her nursing staff. Your physician will need to prescribe needles and syringes in order to aspirate the proper amount of liquid out of the methotrexate vial. You then squirt the specified amount of methotrexate into a glass of juice and drink this once a week. With the liquid form of methotrexate 0.1 cc equals 2.5 mg. If you are on a 7.5 mg dosage once weekly, then you will need to draw 0.3 cc out of the vial and squirt this into your drink. If you are on 20 mg once weekly, the proper dose would be 0.8 cc of liquid methotrexate. Learning how to correctly use liquid methotrexate can save you hundreds of dollars over the course of just six months. The cost of one vial of liquid methotrexate is approximately $45 to $50. Ordinarily you would spend at least this much for just one month of methotrexate tablets. Since the vial has 10 cc of liquid methotrexate in it, this should last for many months. If you are on 0.3 cc each week, for example, then the vial should last you approximately thirty-three weeks. If your insurance carrier does not cover you for either the oral tablets or the liquid methotrexate vial, then another option is to receive intramuscular injections in the physician's office on a weekly basis. Many patients have insurance coverage for intramuscular injections when these are given in a doctor's office. Thus, there are a number of options on how to remain on methotrexate therapy without allowing it to completely bankrupt you.

Using Samples to Help Cut Costs

When pharmaceutical companies come out with new medications, they normally will bring samples to doctors' offices for patient usage. By making these samples available, the companies, of course, hope that doctors will be more inclined to prescribe these medications. From your standpoint, this offers you an inexpensive way to try a new medication without committing to the expense of a full prescription. This also affords you an opportunity to find out whether you will be able to tolerate the new medicine without any adverse side effects. So it is important when your doctor recommends a new medication for you to ask whether there are any samples available that you might try out first. Once you are satisfied that you can truly tolerate a new medication, then you may fill your prescription. This avoids shelling out $50 to $100 for a new drug that then has to be discontinued due to lack of efficacy or side effects

Key Points in Taking Back Control of Your Medication Costs:

1. Don't be duped by well-designed infomercials that are trying to sell you products that are unproven, ineffective, or even potentially dangerous.

2. As with all of the information you receive from television, radio, newspapers, magazines, books, the Internet, or friends and family, you should always run it by your own physician to find out if it truly has merit.

3. If you do not have a history of gastro-intestinal side effects with medications, you may be able to tolerate less expensive over-the-counter or generic forms of NSAIDs to control your arthritis.

4. If you are considered in a "high-risk" group to develop gastro-intestinal complications from NSAIDs, then you may be an excellent candidate for the newer selective COX-2 inhibitor medications.

5. If your rheumatic condition is under excellent control, check with your physician to see if you can reduce your medication costs by being taken off of NSAID therapy.

6. The excellent responses that many patients experience with the new biologic response modifiers (BRMs) may allow them to discontinue or lower their NSAID dosage.

7. Investigate the costs to you of the various forms of methotrexate including tablets, the liquid preparation, or intra-muscular injections and check with your physician to see which form will give you the best outcome at the best price.

8. Take advantage of free medication samples that the pharmaceutical companies supply to your physician for you to take on a trial basis prior to making a significant expenditure on a drug that may not be right for you.

Step 7: Take Back Control of Your Lifestyle

Telltale Signs That Your Lifestyle is Out of Control:

- You are getting less than eight hours of rest each night and are constantly tired.

- You have tried unsuccessfully to quit smoking and continue to smoke at least one pack per day.

- Your diet consists mainly of "junk food" without any significant fruits or vegetables.

- Your diet is poor and yet you don't take any vitamins or calcium supplements.

- You are "burning the candle at both ends" and working long hours followed by partying into the night.

- Your schedule is so hectic that it leaves no time for meditation, prayer, or relaxation.

- You are so busy taking care of your family, that there is little time left to dote upon yourself.

Why You Need to Make Changes in Your Lifestyle Now

Many of my patients are willing to accept my recommendations regarding medications to treat their underlying rheumatic disease, but when it comes to making significant changes in their lifestyle, they find this much more difficult to accomplish. If you do not address lifestyle issues, however, you are putting far too much emphasis and pressure on the efficacy of medications alone. This means that you are losing out on the potential benefits of lifestyle changes, including significant modifications of your diet and exercise program, and your discontinuation of detrimental tobacco and alcohol usage.

Patients who continue to maintain negative lifestyle patterns, which fly in the face of their arthritic conditions, are similar to the diabetic patient who continues to load up on sweets. It is no different than the heart disease patient who continues to eat fatty foods, or the patient with chronic pulmonary disease who continues to smoke. Patients who truly want to get well are those who are willing to make sacrifices and changes that will benefit them the most. Otherwise, in a real sense, you are working against yourself. Not including exercise as part of your regimen allows your muscles to weaken over time. Strong muscles, on the other hand, help protect the joints against damage. If your life is frenetic and out of control and you do not get adequate rest or a proper night's sleep, this may have a negative impact on your immune system. While you may be taking medications designed to help your immune system to battle your disease, your personal habits and life choices may be sabotaging your body's defenses.

Thus, it is time to take stock of your lifestyle. You need to take a good look in the mirror and examine all aspects of your life and see where you can make changes that will be beneficial to you. In subsequent sections in Step 7, we want to help you to address how you can take back control of your lifestyle to improve your arthritis. Do not make the mistake of totally relying on your medication program by itself. Use the knowledge gained in this section combined with your own willpower to make the adjustments in your life that will allow you to take back greater control of your arthritis.

The Importance of Your Diet

Wouldn't it be just great if you could improve or arrest your arthritis by just eliminating certain foods from your diet? This is a very appealing theory to patients, i.e., that something you eat or something in your environment is causing or aggravating your arthritis. You reason that if you could just identify and eliminate certain foods, then you might have a chance at improving. When it comes to actual specific food items, however, this turns out to be a very rare event. Years ago Dr. Richard Panush found a handful of rheumatoid arthritis patients who got worse with particular foods. These foods included dairy products as well as nightshade plants including tomatoes. Obviously, with over two million individuals suffering from rheumatoid arthritis in the United States alone, this turns out to be an extremely unusual association. When patients convey to me that they are experiencing flare-ups every time they eat a certain food, I suggest to them that they eliminate it from their diet to see if it makes a difference. If they are uncertain about the results, they can "re-challenge" themselves with this particular food to verify that it was indeed causing the flare-up and was not just a coincidence.

One rheumatic condition where diet does have a clearer role is gout. Patients with gouty arthritis have excessive levels of serum uric acid. In the vast majority of patients, this really has more to do with a problem excreting the uric acid in the kidneys than it does with the dietary load of purines that are subsequently converted into uric acid. Purines are found in high amounts in organ foods such as liver, kidneys, intestines, and brain. An individual, however, would have to eat an enormous quantity of organ foods in order to elevate the uric acid level appreciably. Another common reason that people develop gout has to do with an excessive intake of alcohol, which I will address in a subsequent section.

Another dietary consideration with rheumatic diseases has to do with the potential for gastrointestinal problems in these patients. Scleroderma patients, for example, may have esophageal involvement with reflux. It would not be advisable for them to be eating extremely spicy or highly acidic foods, which might aggravate this situation. This also could be said of patients who are having gastrointestinal side effects from NSAIDs. These provocative food items should be avoided so as not to exacerbate any gastrointestinal symptoms that may be occurring secondary to medication.

There is evidence that deep-water fish contain a healthy amount of beneficial fatty acids that are anti-inflammatory. Omega-3 fatty acids are particularly high in cod, mackerel, tuna and swordfish. It is recommended that you eat a portion of fish approximately three times a week. There are fish oil tablets available, which could be substituted for eating the fish itself, but these have to be taken in large quantity and they are somewhat odious to swallow. Recent concerns have been aired about the possibility of mercury toxicity from eating too much fish, especially tile fish, swordfish, and tuna. You should check with your own physician regarding how to best balance out the potential benefits of fish consumption with these new revelations about mercury levels.

With what I have told you thus far, you may be wondering why "arthritis cookbooks" exist if there is really no specific recommended diet for arthritis patients across the board. Other than the points that I have made in previous paragraphs, there is no scientific validity for recommending a special "arthritic diet" to everyone. Of course, these types of books sell well because of the public's fervent hope that simple dietary manipulations will lead to marked improvement in their joint symptoms. I wish it were true as well, but unfortunately it has just not proven out in the vast majority of cases. It still may be helpful and healthy to eat a well-balanced diet, not only including the fish meals that I have recommended, but also with adequate meat and vegetables. I mention meat because a number of the rheumatic diseases may be associated with anemia. You may need to have some red meat in your diet to help counteract the anemia. A well-balanced diet should give you the proper amount of "fuel" to fight your arthritis each and every day.

I want to warn you against trying starvation-type diets. In

gout, for example, starvation can actually lead to a potential flare up of your arthritis. Those of you who are using starvation as a means of weight loss should know by now that this isn't a successful means of weight reduction. Oftentimes patients will not only regain the weight that they have previously lost, but will often rebound to a higher weight following a starvation diet. This also could be a problem for those of you who need to take your NSAIDs with food. If you are taking these on an empty stomach to avoid eating, this will put you at greater risk for gastritis or a gastric ulcer. You should, therefore, make sure that you take these with adequate food in your stomach.

Weight-Related Issues

Carrying around an excessive amount of weight for many years certainly can put you at increased risk for developing osteoarthritis (degenerative arthritis) of the lower extremity joints. Over a period of years patients will gradually lose the cartilage in the medial or lateral compartments of the knees. Eventually this leads to a situation called "bone against bone" where there is bony contact leading to significant pain. Obesity can also aggravate low back problems including lumbar disc disease as well as degenerative arthritis of the joints of the lumbar spine. Herniation of the disks, which then can lead to nerve irritation down the leg (sciatica), may be aggravated by excessive weight as well.

It is sometimes difficult to convince an orthopedic surgeon to consider operating on an individual with extreme obesity when it comes to joint replacement of the hips or knees, or low back surgery. This is because these patients tend to have poorer outcomes. There is a higher likelihood of loosening of a prosthesis in the knee when there is excessive weight. The average lifespan of a prosthetic knee replacement is usually from ten to fifteen years. This certainly could be shortened considerably in an extremely overweight individual who would be applying a much greater force to the prosthesis over time.

Excessive weight also may contribute to a higher degree of fatigue and inactivity. Patients who are severely overweight, tend to be the ones who are least likely to exercise. They also may be disinclined to join in aquatic activities because of concern about their appearance in a bathing suit and embarrassment with their weight. If they are experiencing osteoarthritic pain in the hips or knees, then it actually could be detrimental for them to do weight-bearing type exercise as this may serve to accelerate the rate of deterioration of the cartilage of the lower extremity joints. Thus, mapping out an exercise program for the massively overweight individual becomes much more of a challenge than for a slender arthritic patient.

Your excess weight problem should certainly be addressed by your rheumatologist with plans for sensible and gradual weight reduction. This would not only be beneficial for your arthritis, but also is essential for improvement in your general health and well-being. Weight-reduction could decrease your potential risk for the development of diabetes mellitus and hyperlipidemia. It will decrease the likelihood of future heart disease. Therefore losing a significant amount of weight is a "win-win" situation when it comes to arthritis and concerns about your general health.

Unfortunately, the current medication programs available to assist you with weight reduction are somewhat limited and disappointing. A medicine called Xenical (orlistat) prevents the absorption of some of the fat present in your food. Instead of being absorbed, the fat is then excreted in the stools. Unfortunately, this often leads to greasy stools and sometimes the embarrassing development of fecal incontinence (sometimes without warning!). One of the reasons that Xenical may sometimes be effective is that patients may intentionally reduce their fat intake in order to avoid the frightening possibility of having a sudden bowel movement in their pants in a public setting. Reducing the fat intake results in decreased caloric consumption and may lead to weight loss.

A medication called Meridia (sibutramine), which is actually an antidepressant, may reduce body weight by 10 to 15%. Unfortunately, some patients experience side effects with this medication including light-headedness or dizziness. You need to check with your doctor to see if this is an appropriate medication to try in your case.

You need to be careful about over-the-counter products claiming to produce significant weight loss. Some of these products have been shown to contain potentially dangerous stimulants. It is true that you may feel a tremendous amount of energy with these and may even lose weight, but these may be hazardous. They may cause unwanted increases in your blood pressure and could cause potential cardiac complications.

Unfortunately, patients often want a quick fix for their excess weight. Rapid weight loss is usually not sustained and patients will frequently rebound to an even higher weight. Slow weight loss is really the key. Your goal should be to just lose one or two pounds per week maximally. This is best accomplished by changing your dietary habits along with increasing your utilization of calories through increased activity and exercise.

The best way to reduce the calories in your diet is to cut back significantly on the percentage of fat and carbohydrates that you are taking. This means that you should be cutting down on the amount of fried and fatty foods that you eat. If you can avoid bread, potatoes and other starches as well as pure candies and cakes, this will also help. I recommend to my patients that they purchase an inexpensive calorie counter booklet at the check-out counter in the supermarket. Many of them are absolutely surprised and amazed at the calories present in many foods that they are regularly consuming. They are flabbergasted when they see the fat content of some of these items as well. If patients make the switch-over to eating more fish, lean meats, chicken (broiled or baked but not fried), turkey (without the skin or gravy) along with a larger consumption of fruit and vegetables, then they can be successful at reducing their daily caloric intake.

Normally we burn up approximately 1500 calories per day. For every 1000 calories that you burn over and above the calories that you consume, you could expect to lose half a pound. If you burn 2000 calories more than you consume, you can anticipate losing one pound. In this example, you would need to burn up a total of 3500 calories just to lose one pound. This differential between calories consumed and calories burned is an easy mathematical equation for patients to understand and simplifies what it is that you need to do in order to lose weight. Some people are more successful when they monitor their food intake in the form of a diary. It is then possible to count calories to see exactly what one is taking in during a 24-hour period of time. A significant reduction in excessive body weight is a goal well worth the effort. Some patients with low back pain note a resolution or marked decrease in the degree of pain as they drop the pounds. In general, patients with hip and knee pains do better once they have lost a significant amount of weight. You will also feel better overall, and losing this weight could add years to your life.

Should You Rest More, or Less?

Patients with rheumatic diseases are often confused about how much rest they should actually get. Other family members who are not knowledgeable about rheumatic diseases tend to push the arthritic member of the family (often against their will) to do more and more. The family member's intentions may be good, but this kind of advice can be extremely detrimental. Most lay individuals think that the reason that patients get arthritis is that they are not exercising enough. They have no understanding of the immune basis of inflammatory arthritis such as rheumatoid arthritis. Even in the midst of an active flare-up they will still get on a patient's case to try to push them to be more active at a time when they clearly should be less active.

Over thirty years ago, it was often standard practice to hospitalize patients for flare-ups of their rheumatoid arthritis and treat them with bed rest and physical therapy. And guess what happened? Almost all patients would get well once you took them out of their home and work environment and put them at complete rest. This is because inflammatory polyarthritis (including rheumatoid arthritis, ankylosing spondylitis, or psoriatic arthritis) responds better to rest than overuse.

Clearly there is a balance between exercise and rest and the patient needs to know when to increase or decrease one versus the other. When inflammatory arthritis is under excellent control due to the medication regimen, this is clearly an opportunity to gradually increase the level of exercise and the amount of time spent strengthening and conditioning the muscles. On the other hand, if a patient develops active inflammation of the lining of the joints (synovitis) associated with a flare-up, this is the time to cut back considerably on the amount of time devoted to exercise and get a lot more rest. Depending on the severity of the flare-up, this does not automatically mean that an individual has to cut out exercise completely. For example, if it is just a mild flare-up, an individual may want to just do some easy aquatic exercises rather than combining aquatics with any more aggressive land exercises such as walking, jogging or bicycling. Those patients who tend to do the best are the ones who have a clear understanding of how to regulate the amount of time that they rest versus that devoted to their exercise program. Don't be afraid to reduce your exercise if necessary. What you also need to do is educate your family members on when to back off so that they do not pressure you into doing something that is detrimental to your inflammatory arthritis.

Take Back Control of Your Sleep

There are a number of reasons why patients with arthritis and other rheumatic conditions have trouble getting adequate and sustained sleep. Some patients, of course, are in chronic pain that is not well controlled. Painful stimuli from the joints and muscles interfere with the ability to get restful sleep. Clinical research done in sleep laboratories has emphasized the importance of getting what is called restorative sleep. It is a controversial area, but apparently some individuals who have fibromyalgia syndrome often lack this portion of their sleep cycle.

A change in position during the night is often all it takes to stir up arthritic pain and disturb your sleep. Also if patients are in pain and then have to get up to take medication in the middle of the night, it could take a while before they are able to fall back to sleep.

Some medications may interfere with restful sleep. A particular example of this involves corticosteroids, especially when used in higher dosages. This leads to insomnia and makes the average individual feel "hyper." Some other medications may cause nightmares. This is sometimes seen with some of the muscle relaxants. It also can be seen with beta-blockers for those of you taking these for your high blood pressure or cardiac problems.

The worry and anxiety that you feel (we will discuss this further in Step 10) may cause great difficulty in your ability to fall asleep easily. Your mind may be jumping from one concern to another. It is sometimes difficult to prevent yourself from dwelling on all of the worrisome considerations in your life. Once you have actually fallen asleep, your anxious feelings may once again awaken you out of any restful sleep.

Some patients are taking medications that affect the central nervous system during the day with sedating side effects. If this leads to prolonged napping during daytime hours, this can contribute to a reversal of the normal sleep pattern. It would then be more difficult for you to fall asleep at night. In order to get back to a proper sleep pattern, you would need to limit your daytime sleeping to briefer naps, so that you can enjoy a more sustained period of sleep at night.

Some patients with rheumatic diseases may experience hyperirritability. This is seen particularly in systemic lupus erythematosus patients, especially those with central nervous system involvement. A lack of sleep may further aggravate these hyperirritability symptoms.

Many fibromyalgia patients complain of constant fatigue. Fatigue also may be seen in association with rheumatoid arthritis and other forms of inflammatory arthritis, especially at the time of flare-ups. A lack of adequate sleep (consisting of seven to eight hours of rest per night) could further exacerbate the fatigue. If you become more fatigued, you then might not have the energy to do things that you previously enjoyed. This can lead to a sense of frustration for you. Certainly, if you are devoid of any energy, you are less likely to participate in a regular exercise program. Therefore, poor sleep habits could have an indirect impact on your strength and overall conditioning.

There are a number of steps that you can take to help solve your sleep problems. First of all, you do need to recognize that you have a sleep problem (insomnia). You can make changes in your lifestyle to maximize your chances of getting a good night's sleep. Obviously, if you are partying until all hours of the night, instead of trying to get a proper amount of sleep, then you need to make appropriate changes in your schedule. Make sure that you discuss this symptom with your physician so that he or she is aware of it and can make additional recommendations to you. If it is possible for you to avoid medications that are contributing to the insomnia, such as corticosteroids, then this could be extremely helpful. Try some very simple measures at first, such as taking a hot tub bath before trying to fall asleep. Sometimes people find that drinking a warm glass of milk is effective. If there are no contraindications to it, a glass of wine in the evening might help you relax as well.

When it comes to medications for sleep, you may want to try Tylenol PM with your doctor's permission. This consists of acetaminophen along with Benadryl. The Benadryl is an antihistamine and this makes most people feel drowsy. Some individuals may feel somewhat sedated in the morning after taking the Benadryl and this could pose a mild problem for them. Remember to add the quantity of acetaminophen contained in the Tylenol PM to the total calculation of your daily acetaminophen dose. You do not want to exceed 4000 mg of acetaminophen per day.

There are also prescription sleep medications available. One of the more commonly used ones is Ambien. Similar to the after-effects of Tylenol PM, some individuals may feel "hung over" when they get up in the morning. Also make sure that you are not developing any problems with a loss of memory. This can be seen with chronic Ambien use or with higher doses of a number of sleep medications. This is a problem that was more typically seen previously with Halcion. A more recently approved sleep medication, Sonata, is shorter-acting than the Ambien or Halcion. Due to its short half-life, there is less likelihood of feeling sedated when you get up on the morning. Since it is shorter acting, it can also be utilized for those people who tend to wake up at 3 a.m. or 4 a.m. and need something that they can take to get back to sleep for the next several hours without feeling too sedated in the morning.

If it is an overriding sense of anxiety or "panic" that prevents you from falling asleep, then the use of an anti-anxiety medicine such as Xanax (alprazolam) may be effective in not only settling you down, but allowing you to fall asleep. Sometimes antidepressants used at bedtime can also be effective in alleviating your insomnia. Desyrel (trazodone) is probably used as much or more for insomnia as it is for the direct treatment of depression. Elavil (amitriptyline) also is still used at night for this purpose. Some patients with fibromyalgia have found that by taking a muscle relaxant at bedtime, this prevents muscle spasms from keeping them up throughout the night. Thus, a nighttime dose of Flexeril (cyclobenzaprine) or Soma (carisoprodol) can help lead to a restful night's sleep while also relaxing the muscles. Valium (diazepam) is also a muscle relaxant and can be used in low dosages as a helpful adjunct for sleep. Certainly with all of these possible choices, you need to check with your own physician and see whether any of these medications is a reasonable choice in your own situation. I cannot emphasize enough, however, how important it is that you work towards getting seven or eight hours of sleep per night so that you will have sufficient energy to deal with the other steps in this 12 step program to take back control of your arthritis. If you are constantly "dragging around" all of the time and feeling exhausted, you will be less likely to fight back and take back control of your arthritic condition.

Rheumatic Disease: No Butts About It

Everyone has by now been educated regarding the general health risks associated with smoking. The relationship between cigarettes and lung cancer, chronic obstructive pulmonary disease (COPD) and emphysema, as well as heart disease are all well established. Some of you may not, however, be aware of the additional risks of smoking when it comes to rheumatic disorders.

One vascular condition which is worsened by the effects of nicotine is called Raynaud's phenomenon. In this disorder patients may experience extreme coldness of the digits of the fingers and toes associated with white, red, or purple color changes. These symptoms may be triggered by cold temperatures or emotional upset. The digital blood vessels temporarily close down (vasospasm) cutting off circulation to the tips of the fingers and toes. When this process occurs in a patient with a rheumatic disorder such as systemic lupus erythematosus (SLE), scleroderma or rheumatoid arthritis, we call it Raynaud's phenomenon. If the digital vasospasm occurs independently of a rheumatic disease, then it is termed Raynaud's disease. This condition may improve with the discontinuation of smoking. Symptomatic relief can be achieved by wearing gloves and heavy socks and by avoiding cold temperatures. One form of therapy involves the use of calcium channel blockers, which help the blood vessels dilate and thereby improves circulation to the tips of the digits.

There are a number of rheumatic conditions that can be associated with significant lung disease. These tend to be worsened by smoking. Rheumatoid arthritis and scleroderma in particular may have pulmonary manifestations, which can be exacerbated by chronic cigarette use. Prior research has even suggested that the combination of rheumatoid arthritis and smoking induces more severe lung disease than either of these by themselves.

There is also research to indicate that cigarette smoking may at least double the risk of developing rheumatoid arthritis in postmenopausal women. It increases the chances of having a positive rheumatoid factor blood test, which in turn is associated with an increased likelihood of developing rheumatoid arthritis.

Smoking definitely has been shown to have a detrimental effect on blood vessel walls. It is involved in the pathogenesis of a disease called Buerger's disease (thromboangiitis obliterans), which is characterized by blockage of the arteries particularly seen in young male smokers. There is also some evidence to suggest an association between smoking and inflammation of blood vessel walls (vasculitis), such as is occasionally seen in rheumatoid arthritis patients. As the percentage of people smoking has declined, so has the incidence of rheumatoid vasculitis.

Smoking has also been implicated as a risk factor in inducing osteoporosis. Some of this may have to do with a negative effect of nicotine on hormones needed to maintain normal bone mineral density. It should be apparent to you from the above general health risks and musculo-skeletal concerns that it would be best if you did not smoke. If you already have a history of rheumatoid arthritis, systemic lupus erythematosus, scleroderma, Raynaud's phenomenon, vasculitis, or osteoporosis, then you need to speak to your doctor to find successful ways to discontinue this detrimental habit. Treatment options that need to be explored include the use of Nicorette gum, the Nicoderm patch, a medicine called Zyban, and hypnotherapy.

Don't Overindulge with Alcohol

There is mounting evidence that there may be some general health benefits of drinking a glass of an alcoholic beverage on a daily basis. Even as little as half a cup of wine, beer, or hard alcohol several times a week was able to lower the incidence of heart attacks. Mild to moderate amounts of alcohol may be able to prevent strokes, whereas heavy consumption may actually increase the risk. Small amounts of alcohol may decrease the loss of cognitive function and dementia in seniors.

In spite of these potential benefits, there are a number of precautions regarding the use of alcohol in patients with rheumatic disorders. The majority of patients with arthritis are taking an NSAID medication as part of their regimen. The main side effect from NSAIDs involves gastro-intestinal irritation. Patients may develop irritation of the stomach lining (gastritis) or esophagus (esophagitis), an actual ulcer, or even gastro-intestinal bleeding. Excessive alcohol intake can increase the risk of developing these gastro-intestinal complications. In fact, these types of gastrointestinal problems can occur secondary to alcohol even in patients not on NSAIDs. The combination of alcohol and NSAIDs, however, creates an even greater risk for that individual.

Certain DMARD medications have the potential to cause liver inflammation or even significant liver damage. Methotrexate, Arava, and Imuran all require monitoring of liver function tests to make sure that these are not adversely affecting the liver. If you are taking any of these drugs, then you should certainly avoid any alcohol intake. There have been cases of fulminant liver failure with Arava in spite of the doctor following a patient's laboratory tests appropriately. Heavy alcohol just adds to the risk.

Alcohol has been implicated as a precipitating factor in triggering acute attacks of gout. Some patients may "binge" on the weekends and then develop a red, hot, swollen great toe (podagra) on Monday morning. Those individuals with a history of recurrent episodes of gout following heavy drinking should avoid excessive alcohol consumption.

Heavy drinking can have other detrimental effects on rheumatic disease patients. If you are drinking to the point of intoxication, it can interfere with your memory and cognition, and you may forget to take your medicines regularly or in the correct amounts. Excess alcohol can interfere with one's balance. In an elderly individual, who already may have mild balance problems, this can add another layer of risk for falling. Since alcohol is considered one of the risk factors for the development of osteoporosis, these falls could possibly result in a fractured bone. If you have arthritis in the lower extremities, which affects your gait, you need to have a clear head and all of your physical capacities intact in order to avoid an unnecessary fall. With heavy alcohol consumption, it decreases the likelihood of your participating in a regular exercise program. With an unbelievable hangover or a pounding headache, you are not likely to roll out of bed and head straight over to the work-out machines at the local health club.

I certainly would be the last person to want to spoil all of your fun. Life is brief, and you should try to enjoy yourself in spite of your rheumatic disease, but when it comes to alcohol this needs to be done in moderation. If your medications preclude you from imbibing alcohol, then you need to respect this fact and simply accept this as a necessary part of your treatment program. The pleasure you might gain from alcoholic beverages is not worth the risk of some disastrous complication.

Coffee, Tea, Caffeine, and Rheumatic Disease

A large study involving over 18,000 coffee drinkers in Finland concluded that there was an increased risk of the subsequent development of rheumatoid arthritis (RA) in people who drank three or more cups of coffee per day. The Finnish researchers did not distinguish between caffeinated and decaffeinated coffee drinkers. In an even larger study out of the University of Alabama, over 31,000 women were evaluated. In contrast to the Finnish study, they did analyze decaffeinated coffee drinkers separately. They concluded that in people who drank four or more cups of decaffeinated coffee per day, the risk for the development of RA was more than doubled (relative risk of 2.58). On the other hand, women who drank more than three cups of tea per day had a reduced risk of RA (relative risk of 0.39). There was no direct relationship between the intake of caffeine and the subsequent incidence of RA.

Tea may have other medicinal value. Black, green, or oolong tea may have beneficial effects on bone mineral density (BMD). With two cups of tea per day, BMD in the femur was 6.2%

higher than those who did not drink tea regularly. These beneficial effects of tea may be secondary to flavenoids (catechins) and fluoride present in tea.

Tea has been touted as a way to increase the calories an individual burns up in a twenty-four hour period. A major portion of this effect may be actually due to the caffeine in tea as opposed to the flavenoids tea contains.

Caffeine, of course, can be present not only in coffee or tea, but also in sodas. This can have a stimulatory effect on your body. For some of you who are feeling sluggish and fatigued, this may be a welcome boost. It may energize you enough for you to then participate in an exercise program. Caffeine may be detrimental in other individuals by overstimulating them. Those of you struggling with feelings of anxiety may seem even more jittery. If you already have a sleep disorder, the intake of excessive amounts of caffeine may only aggravate your inability to fall asleep and stay asleep. Taking a great deal of caffeine may also lead to a higher level of acidity in your stomach. This may add to the risk of your NSAID medication. You will need to examine your own situation and decide whether you are overdoing it with your caffeine intake. If you are feeling "hyper" or excessively nervous or having problems with getting restful sleep, you may certainly consider cutting back significantly on caffeinated beverages or eliminating your caffeine intake altogether. More research needs to be done to clarify these interrelationships.

Achieving Balance in Your Life

When you watched the juggler perform in the circus when you were a young child, I am sure that many of you never thought that you would end up taking this up professionally during your lifetime. Yet, those of you with significant arthritic problems find yourself doing the juggling act on a daily basis. By that, I mean that you are having to somehow juggle your workload, your home responsibilities, as well as your own personal needs. To me, this is a lot harder than juggling three or four bowling pins. At times you feel as though you are pulled in a thousand different directions. If there are pressing family problems or other ill members in the family, the tendency is to put your own needs aside in order to help those who need it more. This, of course, can be extremely detrimental to your own condition. I have innumerable examples from experiences with my patients in my own practice. For example, a mother whose daughter was suffering with metastatic cancer allowed her own rheumatoid arthritis to progress significantly because she could not devote the time or energy to deal with her own medical problems. I see this frequently when a husband gets ill and my female patients devote themselves exclusively to the spouse's problem leaving no time for their own needs.

Even those of you who do not have a sick family member to deal with also tend to have trouble achieving a proper balance in your life and in your daily schedule. I have had patients tell me that there is just no time to incorporate an exercise program into their daily and weekly schedule. If you are a person who is having problems spending the time required to improve your rheumatic condition, then I suggest that you sit down and chart your daily schedule of activities. You are going to need to modify those expenditures of time that are not helping you to get well. You certainly want to eliminate wasted hours. For example, if you are watching an excessive amount of television instead of exercising, then a change in your priorities is absolutely necessary.

Many patients tell me that they have trouble refusing requests for commitments of their time, for example to volunteer at their church or synagogue, or to help out at their children's school. One of the most important things that you need to do in taking back control of your arthritis is to learn to say "no." You must protect your joints along with your general health and learn to refuse requests for your time that are not in your own best interest. There can, of course, be psychological benefits from volunteering in community activities, but you need to limit these. This certainly needs to take a lower priority than your need for daily exercise.

Some of you lead hectic lives and do not devote any significant time to spiritual issues. It can be extremely beneficial for you to find time to meditate or pray. This may be done at your religious institution or it can be just communing with nature in your neighborhood park. It can be soothing to listen to some relaxing music while meditating in a quiet room at home. This very private time will allow you to relax and for a thirty to sixty minute period feel a sense of control over time and all of the forces that are pulling at you during the rest of the day.

To achieve the balance necessary to regain control of your life, you need to open up communications at home with family members. Then you can make them aware of what you can and cannot do, rather than internalizing all of these feelings and being dragged down by household and work responsibilities. You need to put your foot down and stop the marathon. You need to confront your feelings of helplessness and a sense that you have lost control of your life.

It may be helpful to speak to your employer and make certain that he or she is aware of your medical condition and your needs. Often it will surprise you to learn that your employer actually may be more interested in your health and well-being than you thought and may offer some solutions to dilemmas you face in the workplace. If you sit down and list in order of importance the top priorities necessary to gain a sense of control over your arthritis, this will help you to better plan out your time on a daily basis. Obviously, having understanding family members and a sympathetic boss will be extremely helpful to you as you attempt to rebalance your life.

Key Points in Taking Back Control of Your Lifestyle:

1. Make sure that your diet is appropriate for your particular rheumatic condition.

2. Increase your intake of fish to benefit from the anti-inflammatory effects of the omega-3 fatty acids that they contain.

3. Reduce excessive weight to decrease the symptoms and progression of your arthritis involving the lower extremity joints.

4. Rest your joints during flare-ups, but exercise the muscles and joints when your arthritis is quiescent.

5. Teach family members about the pros and cons of exercise.

6. Get seven to eight hours of restful night's sleep as an essential part of your overall treatment program.

7. Smoking is particularly detrimental in conditions with associated lung involvement such as rheumatoid arthritis, scleroderma, or Raynaud's phenomenon.

8. Nicotine may increase the risk of the development of rheumatoid arthritis and osteoporosis.

9. Heavy alcohol consumption can further add to the gastrointestinal risks of NSAIDs.

10. Excessive alcohol should be avoided in patients on methotrexate, Arava, or Imuran.

11. An excessive intake of alcohol may trigger acute attacks of gout in a susceptible individual.

12. Excessive caffeine may contribute to gastric hyperacidity and aggravate feelings of anxiety.

13. Decaffeinated coffee may increase your risk for the development of rheumatoid arthritis.

14. Black or green tea may have medicinal value leading to stronger bones and a decreased incidence of rheumatoid arthritis.

15. Try to find a way to balance out all of the various forces pulling you in a thousand directions.

16. Prioritize the things in your life that are most important for you to take back control of your arthritis.

Step 8: Take Back Control of Your Work Situation

Telltale Signs That Your Work Situation Is Out of Control:

- Your work hours are excessive and often include significant overtime hours.

- Your chair at work is uncomfortable and does not provide adequate support to your back.

- The temperature where you work is extremely cold and you frequently feel a draft blowing on your neck and upper back.

- You have to walk an extremely long distance to get from your parking place to your workstation.

- You have to stand on your feet for a good part of the workday.

- You are required to climb stairs frequently as part of your job requirements and there are no elevators available to you.

- Your work involves lifting heavy items repetitively and this hurts your joints both while you are doing it as well as afterwards.

- Your supervisor is not sympathetic or supportive of your medical situation and seems to resent the fact that you have physical problems, limitations, and special requirements.

- Your fellow workers resent the fact that you cannot work as hard or as rapidly as they can, and that this, in turn, is creating a greater burden for them.

- Not only is your work physically demanding for you, but the job stress is getting to you as well.

Dilemmas in the Workplace for Arthritis Sufferers

People who develop arthritis face a terrible dilemma when it comes to work. As the disease progresses, it may become increasingly difficult to fulfill the tasks that are requirements of your job description. The easy route might seem to be to just quit and go on disability or welfare, but that could leave you and your family in much worse financial shape. It is also a "catch 22" in that if you leave your job, you may end up losing good insurance coverage that will afford you the type of treatment needed for your arthritis. Also by quitting, you may be giving up pharmaceutical benefits that help pay for medicines that are getting increasingly more expensive and difficult for you to pay for on your own. If your job gives you a feeling of self-esteem and self-worth, you might lose these feelings if you just stay at home and do nothing productive or financially beneficial for yourself or your family.

In spite of some progress that has been made as a result of the Americans With Disabilities Act, the sad fact is that the workplace is not well designed for arthritis sufferers. From the parking lot to your workstation, from the hours to the stress, everything is really stacked against you and often runs counter to your personal health needs. In order for you to begin to take back control of your work situation, we need to address each of these issues and provide you with some viable options to make your "work life" better, which may result in improvement or at least not a worsening of your arthritic disorder. I will begin with a discussion of the physical aspects of performing your job and then later in the chapter will also consider some of the emotional aspects of carrying on gainful employment in the face of arthritis.

A Change in Attitude is Needed

For those of you who drive your car to work, many of you may find that you are forced to park a long distance from the entrance to a large building or plant. For individuals with arthritic involvement of the joints of the lower extremities, this can lead to further wear and tear on these joints. A very long walk could lead to significant fatigue even before you have actually started the workday. Therefore, I strongly recommend that you speak to your personal physician and get the necessary forms completed to apply for a disability placard or license so that you may park adjacent to the facility. If there are not enough disability spaces available to accommodate you, then you need to let management know so that they can increase the number of handicapped parking places. Many of you have not requested this because you are embarrassed by your need for such a convenience. Others are still in a state of denial about their illness and have not yet come to grips with their physical disabilities. Some of you would rather aggravate your pain and the severity of your arthritis than be seen parking in a handicapped space.

If you continue with this self-destructive type of behavior, you will never be able to take control of your arthritis. It is time for you to stop such foolish and detrimental thinking and start dealing with reality. You need help when it comes to the workplace. Instead of being demeaned by others when you ask for assistance, you should be congratulated for showing the courage to be able to drag yourself out of bed each day and go to work. Every workday, in spite of your profound stiffness that may go on for hours, and in spite of pain that may be with you throughout the entire day, you somehow conjure up enough strength to go and do your job. You might really be surprised to find out that many of your co-workers actually greatly admire the courage and fortitude that you demonstrate in just showing up at work and doing a good job in spite of your handicaps.

Assess Your Work Environment

To take back control of your work situation, I would recommend that you take the time to do a complete analysis of every aspect of your job. You need to make a list of all of the things on the job that you feel aggravate your arthritis and then a separate list of those things that could be done to make work life easier for you.

Start with the temperature of your work setting. Is it too damp or cold for you, or are there drafts blowing directly on your body? Most arthritis patients do worse with extremely cold temperatures and feel increased stiffness and pain in the cold. A job that involves being in a cold storage area or in the frozen food section of a store would not be a particularly good type of job for arthritis patients to have. Some patients with Raynaud's phenomenon, which involves spasm of the vessels in the fingers and toes, are readily worsened by cold exposure. Raynaud's phenomenon may occur on its own or in association with other rheumatic conditions like scleroderma, systemic lupus erythematosus, or less commonly rheumatoid arthritis. The cold temperatures may turn the fingers and toes to a blanched white, purple, or red appearance with associated pain in the digits. I advise these patients to wear thin gloves even when they just are passing through the frozen food department at their local supermarket. I certainly would never recommend that they take a job that would continuously expose them to the cold.

Fibromyalgia patients also tend to be very sensitive to the cold. They may end up with severe muscle pain and spasm if exposed to low temperatures, cold air conditioning drafts, or cold wind blowing directly on their muscles. If you are experiencing any of these problems, you need to have the vents re-directed away from you, or have a "diffuser" put on the vent to eliminate any strong draft, or else be moved to a warmer setting in the office. You may have to wear additional clothing such as a light sweater to protect the upper back muscles and neck muscles from tightening up on you.

In recent years, more attention has been paid to ergonomics with a greater understanding of how repetitive work activities affect your health and what can be done to prevent such problems. On your list of things that you feel are detrimental, you need to examine your chair and desk, your computer and keyboard, your lifting requirements, and the rest of your daily tasks. This is necessary in order to appreciate if these might be aggravating your musculo-skeletal problems or at a minimum just making it tougher for you to get through the day.

For those of you with low back conditions, it is important that your chair at work provide good low back support and be comfortable. If you are sitting and working on some type of stool, then it should have not only a proper back support but also a place to rest your feet with the knees in a slightly bent position. Your feet should not dangle in mid-air throughout the day as this may actually put more strain on your low back. If the chair is not soft enough, then you should be allowed to bring a seat cushion to work to reduce pressure on the buttock area. This is particularly an issue for patients with ischial bursitis (over the bones that bear your weight with sitting) or with patients with pain over the tailbone (called coccydynia). People with coccydynia also may need to sit on a medical inner tube, which prevents the tailbone from actually making direct contact with the surface of the seat. Patients with lumbar disc disease or lumbar osteoarthritis, both of which are fairly common disorders, also need to increase their comfort with more attention paid to their low back area. Patients with ankylosing spondylitis, an inflammatory form of arthritis of the spine, tend to be the stiffest and feel the worst in the morning, but then actually may improve and loosen up during the course of the day. All of these conditions, along with others that I have not mentioned, may be aggravated by prolonged sitting on a hard chair with poor lumbar support and without an adequate foot rest (if your feet are not in fact touching the floor).

If you are required to use a keyboard extensively at work, then you must have adequate support for your wrists. If you do not, then you are at risk for developing carpal tunnel syndromes in your hands. The median nerve that supplies the thumb, index, and long finger, runs through a tunnel in your wrist. If the wrist if repeatedly held in a flexed or bent position, then this nerve may get "kinked" and this may lead to numbness and tingling in these same fingers. This condition is often treated with anti-inflammatory medication, local injection into the carpal tunnel with cortisone, and with splinting. If the carpal tunnel sufferer, however, returns to the very same work setting and repeats the same adverse type of repetitive activity, then the condition will re-activate or just become a chronic problem. This may then lead to the need for surgery to alleviate the carpal tunnel symptoms. Although resting wrist splints may be part of the treatment, some patients find it difficult to type with these in place. If you can learn to do this, however, that could also help prevent further long-term problems. If you have arthritis of the wrist or hand joints or recurrent carpal tunnel syndromes, then typing and transcribing jobs may not truly be your best choices as an occupation.

You will see the term "repetitive abuse syndrome" often bandied about when discussing work-related problems. The performance of an occasional activity may not be as detrimental as the repetitious type of physical duties that are required on some jobs. For example, occasionally typing a letter during the course of the day may not lead to the same adverse musculo-skeletal problems that result from typing almost non-stop for eight hours throughout the day. Lifting an occasional object weighing fifteen to twenty pounds may be tolerated, but if this is done all day long it may aggravate a person's arthritis or low back problems.

Fatigue as an Important Issue

Many rheumatic diseases are associated with symptoms of fatigue. This is particularly true of inflammatory forms of arthritis, autoimmune diseases, and fibromyalgia. The total number of hours that a person works, therefore, is an important consideration. In general, it is best if you limit your work hours to an eight-hour day and do not agree to work long overtime hours. You will need to discuss this with your own physician, of course, but most arthritis patients worsen with excessive physical activity and do better with rest. Since keeping a job with a forty-hour workweek may be difficult enough, don't try to push yourself beyond your physical limits. Also, if you have a great deal of morning stiffness, it might behoove you to take a job that starts mid-morning or later when the stiffness has worn off. If you are just getting over a major flare of your arthritis that caused you to miss work, then it may be prudent for you to start back to work slowly and to gradually ease back into your job. For example, you might begin by working just part-time and see how you tolerate your work before expanding back into a forty-hour workweek.

Protecting Your Joints at Work

For those of you with foot or ankle problems in particular, as well as with low back, hip, or knee involvement, it is very important for you to think about the footwear that you are using. Consider the type of floor you are walking on or standing on throughout the day. If you are constantly ambulating on hard concrete surfaces, this could aggravate your low back or the joints of your lower extremities. You need to be permitted to wear cushioned type walking shoes, such as Reeboks, New Balance, Air Nikes, or special nursing type shoes with soft soles. You should not be asked to walk long distances within your facility throughout the day. If your work location is on multiple floors, then there should be an elevator available to you so that you don't have to climb stairs. It would be best, of course, if you worked on carpeted floors to cushion the blow of each step that you take.

Work Risks to Yourself and Others

For those of you with significant arthritis in the upper extremities, it could be dangerous and possibly detrimental to your joints to do heavier manual labor or attempt to operate heavy machinery. It would be difficult for you to anticipate at exactly what moment a sudden severe joint pain might strike you, causing you to lose control of the equipment you were operating. This could put you and other co-workers at risk. Remember that even though your primary disease may involve your joints, you may develop some associated muscle weakness. If your joints are very painful, you may not be using the muscles of your extremities as much while protecting the joints from moving a great deal. Over time, this may "de-condition" your muscles. Therefore, you should try to avoid putting yourself in a situation where you might jeopardize the safety of yourself and others because you cannot be one hundred per cent certain of your ability to perform certain required physical tasks. Also, if you are taking sedating medications to control your pain, this could add to the danger of operating heavy machinery.

Pacing Yourself

It is also important to learn to pace yourself properly. You and you alone are the best person to gauge what you can physically do at any point in time and over an extended period of time. You know what your capacity is as far as your ability to lift a certain weight at any given moment. You also are keenly aware of how much work you can handle on a particular day or over the course of a week or month. With this knowledge, you are best able to decide on a comfortable work rate that will not cause a flare in your rheumatic condition. You need to try to stay within your own comfort zone and not be pushed to work at a pace that is potentially detrimental to you and your joints and muscles.

Dealing with Work Stress

Besides these important physical considerations, there are also emotional factors that need to be explored if you truly plan to take control of your work situation. If you work in a very stressful job, this can aggravate your underlying rheumatic condition. Stress may have a negative effect on your immune system and make you more susceptible to illness in general. Flares in rheumatoid arthritis often occur not just after physical overuse of the joints, but also after increased stress in one's life. A stressful job may contribute to insomnia. If you do not get adequate sleep at night, then your condition may worsen.

Stress at work may be the result of multiple factors. An excessive workload may certainly be important, especially in a person who is somewhat handicapped and has trouble even managing a normal amount of work. You may have the misfortune of working under a supervisor who lacks any compassion for what it is like to work in spite of a physical handicap. This individual may be constantly riding you about your inability to do the job. In some cases, he or she may be trying to coerce you into quitting. In other situations, the supervisor may be simply trying to push you harder. Maybe he or she has the mistaken notion that you are not motivated enough and thinks that by harassing you that this will somehow help. This type of boss lacks the insight to understand that you are already pushing yourself in spite of your condition and your pain. This puts you in the unenviable position of basically being pushed from all sides. You are driving yourself harder so that you won't be in jeopardy of losing your job, while your immediate supervisor is constantly on your back trying to get you to work at a level that potentially could aggravate your illness. The result is a job situation that produces extreme anxiety and possibly depression.

Analyzing your work environment and taking appropriate action is often more complicated than simply concluding whether you are physically capable of performing the tasks required. You definitely should have a meeting with your superiors and make sure that they are totally familiar with your condition and the limitations that you have. A letter from your rheumatologist explaining this in more detail and supporting your desire to continue to hold this particular job may also be helpful. By opening up the channels of communication, you may be able to allay their concerns and correct their erroneous perception that you have an attitude problem. You want them to clearly understand that it is your physical condition that is affecting your work performance.

Making the Necessary Changes

If you have determined that there are certain aspects of your job that you are incapable of handling due to your arthritis, you might suggest to your employer that you are willing to take on more responsibilities in other areas that you can manage more easily. This will reinforce your positive attitude to him and demonstrate your desire to offer your services in ways that you can physically handle. You need to find a satisfactory way that you can contribute to the workplace and continue to be worthy of further employment.

If you are dealing with employers that have no "heart" and are not willing to meet and negotiate with you, it may be best to change jobs in order to avoid further stress. You may want to get yourself an attorney to see if they are in violation of our labor laws. I am not an attorney, but I do know that the Americans With Disabilities Act is designed to protect the handicapped individual from detrimental situations. The courts definitely tend to side with the ill employee over the demands of an unsympathetic boss.

If it's your fellow employees that are giving you heartache because of your absenteeism or your productivity, you need to have a "heart to heart" with them alone or in the presence of an understanding supervisor to set them straight. If in spite of this the situation is still ugly, then you may be forced to find other work or else suffer the physical and emotional consequences of constant stress.

I mentioned earlier how important it is to be able to hold down a job and provide for your family. I have many male patients who completely fall to pieces when they are forced to quit their job due to their arthritis. In some cases, they have been doing heavy work for thirty to forty years and now have to face the fact they are no longer physically able to provide for their families. This is an enormous blow to their egos and frequently leads to significant depression requiring medical treatment. Even women patients will have trouble dealing not only with the financial consequences of being incapable of holding a job, but also with the loss of self-esteem that comes with it.

So if you want to take back control of your work situation, you need to do your homework assignment and make your two lists. You must actively work on all of the improvements you have listed in your second column. Open up the channels of communications between you and your fellow workers and you and your boss. Make sure that everybody truly understands what you are going through each and every workday. Let them know how important it is for you to keep that job. Make certain that they know that you are giving your maximal effort, but that you are limited by your rheumatic condition or by the side effects of the medications that you must take in order to control it. Try to convince them of the important changes that can be made to better accommodate you and your musculo-skeletal problems. They need to appreciate that a happier, more satisfied employee, who is in less pain, will be a more productive worker. That worker can then subsequently make significant contributions to their business.

Key Points in Taking Back Control of Your Work Situation:

1. Do your own job analysis of all of the aggravating factors on the job and list how these could be eliminated or improved.

2. Address the physical considerations of the workplace including such things as your parking spot, your chair and desk, the ambient temperature and drafts, lifting requirements and other physical demands of your job (including standing, walking, operating heavy equipment, repetitive typing, or climbing stairs).

3. Avoid working excessively long hours or taking on an unreasonable workload.

4. Identify areas of stress on your job and work towards reducing or eliminating them.

5. Communicate to your fellow workers as well as to your supervisors about the nature of your condition and what limitations it imposes on you.

6. Try to get your supervisor to make the physical accommodations that would make your "work-life" easier for you. Let your boss know that you truly value your job and that you are giving a maximal effort, but that you are unfortunate enough to have to deal with the pain and physical handicaps from your rheumatic condition.

Step 9: Take Back Control of Your Exercise Program

Telltale Signs That You Have Lost Control of Your Exercise Regimen:

- By the time you think about exercising, you are too fatigued to actually do it.

- Every time you attempt to exercise, you start out too enthusiastically and then subsequently experience a flare-up in your arthritis.

- When you develop musculo-skeletal pain while exercising, you ignore this symptom and push yourself even harder to overcome the pain.

- When you exercise, you tend to jump right in and start without any warm-up period or stretching beforehand.

- You have tried lifting weights but this has led to flare-ups of arthritis in your hand and wrist joints.

- Your idea of exercise is putting up a fence, repairing the roof, or trimming the trees.

- You get bored doing the same exercises every day all by yourself.

Don't Start Off Wrong

A great many patients who finally decide to take the plunge and start an exercise program (whether to combat arthritis or just for general health purposes), frequently make numerous errors at the onset. Some of these mistakes are potentially dangerous in that they can lead to serious injuries or at a minimum a setback in your medical status and condition. The first mistake that patients make is that often they do not discuss their exercise plans with their own physician. The first question that needs answering is whether they should even be participating in an exercise program at that point in time in terms of their medical condition. Then there needs to be some discussion about which particular exercises should be performed including their duration and frequency. The doctor should list any specific restrictions and advise the patient on any warning signs to look for in order to know whether they should back off or discontinue their exercise.

Often patients forget that they need to warm up before getting started into the "meat" of their exercise regimen. I cannot overemphasize the need to mildly stretch your muscles before you start going "full tilt." If you start off from a cold start, you may increase the likelihood of injuring yourself. On the other hand, if you overstretch before you are warmed up you can also injure the muscles. This is one reason more prolonged stretching of the muscles should probably be done in the middle or at the end of your exercise session—after you are limbered up.

Another mistake patients make is that they don't adjust the level of exercise to their own capacity. For example, the pace that they set on the treadmill is too rapid or the tension on an exercise machine too great. The patient often tries to push himself or herself too hard and too fast incorrectly assuming that more is better. When it comes to exercise, however, slow and gradual is actually better and safer.

Frequently, patients also start off with too prolonged a period of exercise. They begin by pushing themselves to try to exercise for one hour or more. After all, they reason, there have been a lot of months and years without exercise to make up for. Also, many patients perform too many repetitions with each exercise right off the bat. These same patients will also try to exercise through the pain. They tend to ignore the body's signals that they have overdone it.

The result of overdoing it right out of the gate is the possibility of developing severe muscle pain or spasm and "stirring up" your joint pain. Even following just one extremely prolonged and far too difficult an exercise session, an individual may end up hurting, as well as being incapacitated and discouraged. This person may then swear off subsequent exercise based on the fact that it is too painful to do and because it has led to a flare-up in their other musculo-skeletal symptoms. It will take some re-educating and coercion to get this person back into a proper exercise program. Therefore, instead of starting off and making all of these mistakes at the onset that leave you with a negative attitude about exercise, you need to start off in a proper manner. This encourages you to commit to a long-term exercise program.

Start off by discussing exercise with your rheumatologist. Make certain that he or she feels it is appropriate for you to do this based on your general medical condition as well as your arthritis. Decide which type of exercise is best for you, i.e., which approach is going to be the most effective with the least risk of harming you in any way. Most eighty-year-old women, for example, should be doing mild walking and aquatics and not heavy training with weights or exercise machines.

Speak to your doctor about the length of time he or she recommends that you exercise. When you are first starting out in an exercise program, your initial session should probably last a total of 20 to 30 minutes. Once you have mastered this successfully over a two to four week period, you can then advance up to 45 minutes. Then after an equal period, advance to one hour exercise sessions if tolerated.

Always begin at the lowest degree of difficulty. As I previously stated, if you are using a treadmill set the machine on zero degrees of elevation and start off with a slow speed to see if you can handle this easily. If you are doing aquatic exercises, start off with no more than five to ten repetitions for each exercise so as not to overwork your muscles too abruptly. If you are using a stationary bicycle, set the tension at the lowest possible setting so you can pedal freely without any resistance.

If you start feeling pain either in one particular part of your body or in multiple areas, then you should stop what you are doing and rest. If your pain is localized to a specific joint, you may have performed an exercise that puts too much stress on that joint. You then need to let that joint recover over a period of days or weeks. Avoid repeating that same exercise or simply back off on the number of repetitions or length of time of that particular exercise. This will help to avoid reproducing similar pain in that joint in the future. Learn to respect these painful messages. Use these painful signals as an early alert warning system. Do not attempt to exercise through the pain. You need to back off or you may end up hurting yourself rather than helping yourself.

Therefore, the way you initially begin an exercise regimen is extremely important. If you start off incorrectly you risk harming yourself and doing damage to your muscles and/or joints. By overdoing it at the onset, you may end up with self-induced problems that will discourage you from future participation in an exercise program that you so desperately need.

Understanding the Difference Between Abuse and Therapeutic Exercise

Patients often confuse strenuous physical activity at work or the performance of heavy household tasks with a proper therapeutic exercise program. What many patients describe to me as "their exercise" would be better characterized as "abuse." Down here in Texas, I have a number of patients who do a great deal of ranching and farming. They frequently are required to lift 100-pound bags of feed or heavy sacks of fertilizer. I have other patients who are long-haul truck-drivers, who repetitively lift 50 to 100 pounds or more, and then come and ask me to prescribe medication to help alleviate their pain and joint swelling. This uncontrolled repetitive type of lifting is truly abusive. What I recommend for arthritis patients is a much more controlled form of exercise. The weight and resistance during each exercise should be mild and the repetitions and time span short enough to avoid injury. So when I recommend to you to take back control of your exercise (Step 9) in order to take back control of your arthritis, don't misinterpret this by substituting abusive physical labor instead of a physician-supervised exercise program.

The Goals and Benefits of Exercise for Arthritis Patients

It is important to establish with your physician what goals you are trying to reach with an exercise program. Some patients get so involved with their exercise and do it with such vigor that I sometimes think that they are contemplating qualifying for the next Olympics. My own objectives for my patients tend to be far less lofty. First of all, I am interested in the patient's general conditioning. There are significant cardiovascular and pulmonary benefits to a regular exercise regimen. As a physician I am interested in my patient's general health as well as his or her musculo-skeletal status.

Patients need to understand the beneficial effects of stretching and strengthening the muscles. Patients need to work on building and maintaining good muscle tone throughout the body. We don't want muscles to weaken or get flaccid due to lack of use. Patients also need to preserve a maximum range of motion in the joints. You definitely need to make every effort not to lose any of the motion that you currently have.

Regular exercise will help combat feelings of fatigue that frequently are associated with rheumatic disorders. Exercise may certainly help increase your stamina. During exercise, endorphins are released in the brain. These actually can serve to decrease your degree of pain. Thus, exercise can be a "natural" kind of pain reliever if you do not overdo it. Patients who exercise regularly may often feel increased self-esteem and self-worth. These are some of the psychological benefits to exercise in addition to the many physical rewards that you can expect to achieve.

Don't Fall Victim to Boredom When Exercising

Many arthritis suffers start out with a lot of enthusiasm when they first start an exercise program. Unfortunately, a great many individuals drop out after even a brief period of time due to boredom. If you are simply doing the same type of exercise in a repetitive and monotonous way, then it is highly likely that you will lose interest quickly.

It is important to vary the type of exercise that you are doing as part of each exercise session. On certain days you can concentrate more on muscle toning and strengthening. This could be alternated with days when you simply do aquatic therapy. On other days you may do aerobic land exercises or just some walking. By changing your regimen, you add variety to your exercise program, which sustains your interest.

If you are specifically doing aquatic therapy, then you may want to vary your exercises by choosing from a larger menu of choices. On our *Take Back Control of Your Arthritis: Basic Aquatic Exercises* and our *Take Back Control of Your Arthritis: Advanced Aquatic Exercises* videos, there are thirty different types of exercises from which to choose. You might select anywhere from ten to fifteen of these to do during one session. Each of these video programs comes with a laminated poolside guide so that you can take these with you to the pool and select different ones each time that you exercise. These programs are available at www.ArthritisMall.com or by telephone at 1-800-980-MALL (6255).

Some people find themselves to be less motivated when they are exercising by themselves. They tend to do significantly better as part of a group or a class. This may consist of a group of friends or just other folks in the same physical shape or with similar medical conditions. Certainly, the presence of other arthritis patients in your class pushing themselves to exercise and get well can help motivate you to do the same.

If you are musically inclined, then you certainly want to think about using a headset with a tape recorder or CD player when you are exercising on dry land. Some of you love your radio talk shows and could certainly learn to exercise while listening to your favorite talk show host. Not only will you be mentally stimulated by the provocative conversation, but you will be improving your muscle strength and maintaining your joint motion simultaneously. If you feel that you are depressed, then listening to comedy tapes or CDs might lighten things up. Try starting out with some of the Bill Cosby classics. This will cheer you up while you are pushing yourself through your exercise program.

If you are in an occupation where you need to catch up with educational or instructional tapes, what better opportunity is there then to do this while exercising! I really enjoy walking on the treadmill while listening to tapes from my arthritis meetings. This helps pass the time and forces me to concentrate on the information on the tape rather than on the exercise itself.

A large number of people enjoy watching T.V. while exercising. Some individuals will use a particular program as a motivating factor. My wife, for example, exercises to her favorite soap opera, *Guiding Light*. Thus, she knows that she is going to get her one-hour of exercise each weekday by combining the exercise with a program that she enjoys. Patients with arthritis who are sports fanatics might learn to watch particular sports events during their exercise program instead of becoming "couch potatoes." For example, walking on the treadmill or using a stationary bicycle while watching a golf tournament on the weekends is a great way to take advantage of these precious hours.

All of these techniques that I have suggested are ways of distracting you from the boredom of repetitive exercise by not doing exactly the same type of exercise every single day. You are more likely to persist with an exercise program that is varied. Remember that variety, after all, is "the spice of life." By using some form of entertainment, this will help pass the time away. It might actually encourage you to look forward to your exercise when it is combined with a particular television or radio program, tape, CD, or DVD. The key here is to try to make your exercise fun as well as beneficial.

Setting Exercise Goals to Increase Your Motivation

When you exercise aimlessly without specific targets in mind, this can not only create boredom but can convince you to end your exercise session prematurely. There are a number of ways you can set goals that will stimulate you to exercise effectively and for longer periods of time.

You can simply use time as an endpoint. For example, if you know that you are going to be on the treadmill for thirty minutes according to the clock, then you are likely to complete your objective. You could use the timing at the beginning and end of a T.V. or radio show that runs thirty to sixty minutes in length. You could also decide that you are going to exercise during the second half of a basketball or football game or during a thirty or sixty minute evening news show. Another way to go about this is to decide that you are going to get through a defined set of exercises. For example, if you are doing aquatic exercises, you might tell yourself that once you have finished performing fifteen of these exercises, you will have successfully completed that exercise session. If you are just starting out on an exercise regimen, you might start out gently with just five exercises. Then each week, add one more exercise until eventually you have worked up to a total of fifteen exercises. This is particularly useful when doing aquatics, so that you gradually build up your endurance. In 1996, the Surgeon General of the United States had recommended thirty minutes of daily exercise for everyone. Then in September of 2002, the Institute of Medicine in Washington, D.C. suggested raising this requirement to one hour daily, but included chores around the house and any other moderate physical activity as contributing towards this sixty-minute goal. So everyone needs to focus on setting aside up to one hour per day to get proper exercise—not just arthritis patients.

You can also vary the difficulty of your exercise program based on the number of repetitions or distances involved. For example, if you are doing "water walking" as one of your aquatic exercises, you might start by walking just one half of the length of the pool. The next week you might increase to walking three quarters of the length of the pool. By the third week, you can advance up to one full length of the pool. You then can decide to increase gradually even beyond that. If you are treading water in the pool, you may start off by only doing this for thirty seconds. Then gradually try to build up to one to two minutes or more. If you are doing exercises at home such as leg lifts, you can start off with three lifts on each side and then over a period of weeks gradually advance up to ten to twenty leg lifts per side. Apply this same approach to your other exercises as well.

You can also try to add resistance by using weights to gradually make your exercise more demanding. If you are doing straight-leg-raises while in bed, then start off by just learning to lift your leg vertically off of the bed. Then you can make this somewhat more challenging by adding one-pound ankle weights. Once you are able to tolerate this, you can then proceed to two-pound weights. You should always back off if you find the increased weight or resistance too strenuous or too painful. Also with this particular type of exercise, you need to ease off if this bothers your lower back muscles.

If you enjoy walking on a treadmill, then try starting off without any elevation at a slow speed. Eventually you can begin adding one degree of elevation each week and see what you can comfortably tolerate. The elevation increases would not be recommended for individuals who have balance problems. You also can gradually try to build up your speed along with the elevation changes. Remember, however, that walking at a reasonable speed without any elevation is still very good exercise. Don't overpush yourself.

If you enjoy walking outdoors or in a mall, you can start off by walking one quarter of a mile and see how you tolerate this. Then you can advance over a period of several weeks up to one half a mile. Once you have conquered this, you could increase to a distance of one mile. You should always back down if you start feeling pain during or immediately following your exercise or within the first twenty-four hours after performing this exercise.

By setting goals in terms of the time you spend on a particular exercise or the difficulty of the exercise, you can motivate yourself to strengthen your muscles even further. Setting goals will also prevent you from getting bored and giving up on your exercise program altogether. Since exercise is such an important step in taking back control of your arthritis. I encourage you to try all of these different techniques to make exercise an integral part of your daily regimen.

Where Do Personal Trainers and Physical Therapists Fit In?

Although it is not essential, some of you may want to look into having a personal trainer to help provide you with some additional expertise and guidance. You may feel that the trainer can provide you with additional motivation in order to meet your exercise goals.

When you are trying to choose a personal trainer, find out if he or she is "nationally certified." You should inquire as to what prior experience he or she has had dealing specifically with arthritis patients. Obviously it would be best to find someone who understands the pain, limitations, and risks associated with exercise in the arthritic individual. The expense of a trainer can add up over time, so before you commit financially to a long-term arrangement, try one or two trial sessions to see if the trainer is meeting your needs and actually listening to your feedback. Some trainers may be so gung-ho in trying to get you to push yourself harder, that they may ignore or minimize your complaints of exercise-induced pain. This may lead to injury or a flare of your arthritis. Try to find someone who respects your symptoms and is a good listener and communicator.

If you are not looking for a general conditioning and strengthening program, but instead have more specific problems with particular joints, then you may actually need the expertise of a physical therapist. The therapist has been educated in handling musculo-skeletal disorders. Typically, before any exercising of joints takes place, modalities such as hot packs or ultrasound are utilized to warm up the surrounding tissues. This will allow for a fuller range of motion in the joint. Physical therapy is usually covered by most insurance carriers, whereas a trainer is not. There is often a limitation, however, to the number of physical therapy sessions that the insurance company will cover annually. Rheumatologists will commonly order a "course" of treatment over a one-month period to treat an acute problem. Working with a physical therapist, therefore, is not something that can usually be done on a constant or long-term basis. Your physician will be able to best advise you on whether or not physical therapy is indicated in your case. If it is, your doctor will actually write a prescription for these treatments. Your rheumatologist will know where to send you to receive the best physical therapy in your area.

Stretch First to Avoid Injury

As I have already stated, when you exercise, it is important to try to stretch your muscles and limber them up before you start. By gently stretching your muscles first, you can avoid straining them as well as injuring any other of your musculoskeletal tissues. If you lean forward against a wall with your legs stretched out behind you, you can perform calf or leg stretches. Stretch your arms upwards over your head, then hold them out in front of you, next to your side, and finally behind you in order to limber up the upper extremity muscles. Five minutes of stretching may go a long way to avoid more serious injury once you have started into your heavier exercise program. It is important for you to perform stretches that you can easily tolerate based on your own rheumatologic condition. Do not try to imitate others, who may be far more limber than you are or whose arthritis is not as severe. Respect the pain and don't overstretch. Stretches are often most helpful when they are done slowly and held for a thirty-second interval. Try to avoid "bouncing" the leg in order to stretch your calf muscles. This just creates very short, sharp stretches and these are not as beneficial as more prolonged slower stretches.

Yoga exercises may be extremely beneficial for improving your flexibility, as long as you don't overdo it. Although it has its original roots in the Hindu religion, yoga has been popularized as an excellent way to combine musculo-skeletal conditioning and stretching with meditation. Some forms of yoga, such as Kundalini yoga include chanting along with the exercising. Hatha yoga is the type of yoga class that you will most commonly see offered. A series of poses (asanas) are performed, and this is tied in with your breathing. During the holding of the pose, you have the opportunity to meditate simultaneously. The combination of the physical and mental aspects of yoga is part of its great appeal. You do need to be warned, however, not to push yourself beyond your own capacity. If you feel any pain, you need to stop immediately. Don't look at other people in the class who may have been doing yoga for years and try to instantaneously imitate them.

Make certain, first of all, that your physician approves of yoga in your particular case. Then start off very slowly and allow yourself to build up to more difficult and more sustained poses over many weeks or months. Don't ever stop listening to the feedback that you get from your own body.

Why Aquatic Therapy is the Best

In my professional opinion, aquatic therapy overall is still the best therapeutic type of exercise for arthritis patients. There is a natural therapeutic benefit of water flowing against the outer body. This may actually help diminish some of the pain you are feeling. Water allows you to easily move your joints through a full range of motion. The buoyancy of water means that you only have to support a small percentage of your total body weight while you are exercising. At the same time, water provides a significantly higher resistance than air. Therefore your muscles get a much better workout than they would on dry land. There are also cardiovascular and pulmonary advantages to aquatic exercise with potential benefits to your circulation and lung capacity.

You can still participate in aquatic exercises even if you are not an accomplished swimmer. If you are a person who does not know how to swim at all or is afraid of the water, you can wear a buoyancy belt or life-jacket to keep your head and neck above water and make you feel more secure.

There are special aquatic exercise pools that are heated to a temperature of 92 degrees. This is an extremely comfortable temperature for patients with arthritis. For an individual who is interested in a more aggressive conditioning program including swimming laps, then an 84-degree temperature pool would be preferable.

Aquatic therapy is also helpful for those patients who are trying to work on improving their balance and coordination. If you fall to one side in the pool while practicing your balancing exercises, the consequences are that you get a little wet as you fall into the water. If you were to fall while exercising on dry land, you could potentially injure your hip if you landed on a hard surface. Thus, aquatic exercise has many advantages for patients afflicted with arthritis. For all of the reasons delineated above, it is the preferred form of exercise for arthritis.

Precautions and Safety Issues with Aquatic Exercise

Certainly before you embark on an aquatic exercise program, it is important to check with your own physician and see if this is indicated in your case. If you have cardiovascular or pulmonary problems or even high or low blood pressure, aquatics may pose some additional risks for you. It is important, therefore, to gain the approval of your physician before you enter an aquatics program.

If you have a skin rash or any open wounds, it is probably best to avoid the water until these are resolved. This will also help protect others who are in the pool. If you have a urinary catheter or a colostomy bag in place or are suffering from bowel or bladder incontinence, then you would not be a good candidate for pool therapy. If you have a soft cast on an extremity, it is not advisable to get it wet. If this cannot be adequately covered and sealed while you are in the water, then it would be best that you wait until the cast has been removed before you start back into your aquatics therapy program.

There are some safety issues that are important when it comes to performing aquatic exercises. You need to always remember that tile surfaces surrounding most pools are slippery when wet. You need to use extreme caution, therefore, when getting in or out of the pool.

You should be careful about overdoing it. As I have previously pointed out, the resistance of water is much greater than that of air. It is easy to be deceived as to how much you have actually exerted yourself during your aquatics exercise. Since aquatics can be extremely fatiguing, you need to start off with fewer repetitions and a shorter time span in the pool. Then you may build up the length and difficulty of your exercise gradually over weeks or months.

Ironically, even though there is lots of water surrounding you while you are doing pool exercises, you may still become dehydrated. It is a good idea to bring a plastic container of water with you to re-hydrate yourself. You do not want to bring any glass items into the pool area. If these were to break, this would pose a hazard for you and other patients.

At the outset, you should try not to swim by yourself. If a problem such as a severe muscle cramp were to develop, you would not have anybody around to assist you. Swimming as part of a group or class provides you with physical and emotional support. You may derive benefit from your social interactions with your classmates. They may provide you with positive reinforcement and share their insights into how they are coping with their own rheumatic conditions.

If you are a person who is embarrassed by your physical appearance in a bathing suit, then you can simply wear a tee shirt over the outside of your bathing suit. There is no absolute requirement that you wear a bathing suit during your pool exercise program. You can wear some other exercise outfit if you prefer, but try to avoid any clothing that gets extremely heavy when wet. This could make it more difficult for you to perform your exercises. During the wintertime, make sure that you dry off well before you venture out of the warmth of the pool area into colder outdoor temperatures.

There is definitely a lot of effort involved in going to a pool, changing into a bathing suit, exercising, then showering, drying off and changing back into your street clothes. Some people will use all of this expenditure of energy as an excuse not to bother with an aquatics program. I want to encourage as many as you as possible to try to overcome the resistance that you may feel towards aquatic therapy because of the huge benefits that it provides to patients afflicted with arthritis.

ArthritisCentral.com has created two comprehensive video programs on aquatic therapy for arthritis patients. We have included a discussion of its advantages, precautions, and safety issues on each program. Each video offers you a set of fifteen separate types of aquatic exercises to perform as part of your overall program. We have filmed these on dry land, from above water, and under water. This makes it extremely easy for you to understand how to perform each of these thirty exercises. Once you have studied and mastered these at home, you can bring your laminated poolside guide with you and select different exercises to perform each time that you go to the pool. By varying your aquatic exercise, it will make it much more interesting for you. It will help avoid the boredom that might set in if you were to always do the same aquatic exercise routine each time that you went to the pool.

We decided that it might be beneficial and fun to combine the benefits of aquatic exercise with Tai Chi. *Take Back Control of Your Arthritis with Aquatic Tai Chi* is the first physician supervised program merging these two excellent forms of exercise. This program has been a big hit with a number of my patients. Remember that it is very important not to get bored with your exercise regimen. Doing aquatic Tai Chi once or twice a week will add some variety to your exercise schedule. You may obtain more information about this program at ArthritisMall.com or by calling 1-800-980-MALL (6255).

Walking Works

Enthusiasm for exercising to improve one's general health or to combat arthritis has contributed to the proliferation of health clubs across the country. Most of these offer great workout equipment as well as lots of very challenging classes (often too difficult for the average arthritis patient). If you are looking for a less expensive alternative that can be done at your convenience, then look no further than your own two feet. Walking is an absolutely excellent form of exercise for arthritis sufferers.

It is important that you have comfortable footwear, which offers you adequate support. If you have any balance problems whatsoever, then I recommend that you carry a walking stick or cane to give you more confidence and protect you from any unnecessary falls. Try to choose a flat, even surface. A local high school or university track may actually have a special softer surface, which will make it easier on your lower extremities. Start off with a thirty-minute walk and then gradually increase your total time up to one-hour or more as tolerated over several weeks or months.

There are lots of interesting places to walk that will help prevent boredom. These special places include local parks or the zoo. See if there is a nature trail in your area. In a hot climate like we have in Texas, the indoor malls are an excellent place to walk. The air-conditioned environment will help prevent you from getting overheated and excessively dehydrated.

Regarding the issue of dehydration, you should either carry a bottle of water with you or be aware of where you can stop along the way to drink. If you are feeling at all light-headed or "woozy," you should stop immediately and start taking in fluids. Check with your own physician and make sure that the exercise that you are doing is advisable with your medical condition. There is more general information available about walking at a website here in my own backyard in Texas at the American Volkssport Association. You may find them at www.ava.org or at 1-800-830-WALK.

Weightlifting and Weight-Training Exercises

Keeping your muscles strong is an important goal of any arthritis exercise program. Strong muscles can help reduce pressure on the joints by absorbing some of the force that would ordinarily be applied to them. Yet weightlifting and other weight-training exercise still remain somewhat controversial.

This controversy can be explained in part by what people mean when they describe weight-training exercises. Most individuals usually have the image of some 250-pound Olympian hulk jerking a 400-pound weight into the air. Extremely heavy weightlifting, however, may result in injury to the arthritic individual. Recently, other concerns have been raised as well regarding general health risks with trying to lift heavy loads. One such concern is regarding the potential to rupture a blood vessel at a point of weakness in the wall (a ruptured aneurysm), which could result in a stroke. Another worry is about marked elevations of blood pressure that may occur during the actual lifting itself as an individual is straining maximally. Therefore, avoiding heavy weights seems safer. It has been suggested that not even "healthy" individuals try to bench press more than half of their body weight. It has also been recommended that an individual not exceed weights that can comfortably be lifted sixty times (with four sets of fifteen lifts each).

The tight gripping that is required in order to lift free weights may aggravate the joints in the hands and wrists. This is particularly problematic in patients with inflammatory arthritis (e.g., rheumatoid arthritis). Also lifting heavier free weights while in the standing position can put undue stress on the low back. This may lead to low back pain with muscle strain and spasm. If the weights are extremely heavy, this can even result in damage to the lumbar discs with possible disc herniation.

On the plus side there is some evidence that the addition of weight-training exercise to an aerobic exercise program further decreases the risk of heart disease. Even just thirty or more minutes per week is all that is required to achieve this benefit.

Also on a positive note, there is research to demonstrate that the addition of weight-training exercises can help reduce pain and improve function. This is particularly true when one strengthens the anterior thigh muscles (quadriceps), which help support the knee. This results in a decrease in perceived knee pain and an improvement in walking, navigating stairs, rising from a seated position, and standing. Individuals with stronger muscles find that they can better deal with activities of daily living.

Many arthritis patients avoid muscle building and strengthening exercises because they are in pain as a result of the destructive process in their joints. If the muscles that support the joint are permitted to weaken further, then this may actually result in even more stress on that joint, resulting in further damage. Therefore some type of muscle strengthening program is beneficial, if it is not excessive or abusive.

As with any exercise, I would first recommend that you get approval from your own physician, who is familiar with your medical condition. I recommend to my patients that they start off gently and only advance to greater resistance with increased weights very gradually. If they experience any significant pain, then they should back off to the next lower weight and see if they can tolerate this. One, two, and five-pound dumbbells are available at any large sporting goods store.

You may wish to add weightlifting or weight-resistance type exercises to your workout regimen once or twice a week. On other days, you can do your aquatics, walking, Tai Chi, or aquatic Tai Chi. Mixing up your regimen will keep you from getting bored. Many health clubs have added what are termed "hybrid" classes, where strengthening types of exercise are merged with cardiovascular or aerobic types of activity. Flexibility and stretching exercises may also be thrown into the mix. If you don't belong to a health club, you can accomplish the same goal by just varying the type of exercise on your own. Using weights to build muscle in an arthritic individual can be beneficial if done in moderation. It is very important, however, to listen to your body and back off if you are feeling pain.

Don't Forget to Work on Your Balance

As many of us get on in years, we sometimes have more difficulty with our sense of balance. This can put us at a significant risk of falling. One inopportune fall could lead to a fractured hip. This can often be a devastating and even fatal medical event with a 20% overall mortality associated with it. Twenty-five per cent of people who incur a hip fracture never regain their former physical function. Therefore, avoiding a hip fracture is extremely important, especially for our senior citizens.

Exercises to improve your balance, which might help avoid a bad fall and subsequent fracture, can actually be done simply in your home. If you are having problems with your sense of balance, you should only try these recommended exercises when there is at least one or possibly two people at your side to assist you.

They will be able to catch you if you are unsteady or start to fall. Start your exercise by standing in an open doorway. Grab each side of the doorframe with one of your hands and hold on tight. Then raise one leg and practice balancing on the opposite leg to the count of ten. Switch legs and now try to bear your weight on the opposite leg. Another way to perform this exercise is to turn two chairs back to back. Then step in between the chairs and hold on to the tops of the backs of the chairs with each hand. Practice balancing on one leg to the count of ten and then switch to the other leg. After you have been doing this for some time, you may then extend the length of time that you balance on each leg. Training yourself in this manner will hopefully not only strengthen your legs, but also improve your sense of balance and help you avoid the consequences of a nasty fall.

One of the best types of exercise to build balance is Tai Chi. Originally this was developed as a form of martial arts, but now has been transformed as a set of exercises that can help arthritis patients. On our video, *Take Back Control of Your Arthritis with Texas Tai Chi*, we have simplified Tai Chi and extracted moves from standard Tai Chi sets of exercise. It is excellent for stretching, strengthening, and conditioning the muscles, as well as for improving your balance. (See ArthritisMall.com for more information.)

Key Points in Taking Back Control of Your Exercise:

1. Check with your physician before undertaking any exercise program.

2. Find out if your doctor has any restrictions or special instructions for you.

3. Start off slowly and only very gradually increase the duration and difficulty of your exercise regimen.

4. Always respect the pain and back off or stop if you feel significant discomfort.

5. Perform therapeutic exercise and avoid abusive activities that are detrimental to your joints.

6. Vary your program to avoid the monotony and boredom of repeating the same exercise incessantly.

7. Establish new exercise goals by increasing the time, distance, or repetitions to motivate you.

8. Do mild stretching before you get started, and then do greater stretching only when you are warmed up.

9. Aquatic therapy, the best exercise for arthritis patients, should become part of your exercise regimen.

10. Walking in proper footwear on a flat, even surface can be an excellent and inexpensive way to exercise.

11. Weight-training to strengthen muscles may be beneficial if done in moderation.

12. Exercises such as Tai Chi, which improve balance, may help avoid unnecessary falls.

Step 10: Take Back Control of Your Emotions

Telltale Signs That Your Emotional State is Out of Control:

- You feel that your arthritis will never get better and you feel hopeless about your situation.

- You find yourself crying or teary-eyed throughout the day, even at times when you are not physically in pain.

- You wonder if God is punishing you for some unclear reason by afflicting you with your arthritic condition.

- You feel very anxious and nervous about what is happening to you and what will become of you in the future.

- You are overwhelmed by stress and guilt about your inability or difficulty in performing your duties as a spouse and parent.

- You feel a great deal of anxiety about whether you will be able to keep your job due to your work limitations, and if you can't you wonder how you will be able to afford the medical costs of your treatment.

- You lie awake each night and cannot fall asleep as you worry about your disease, job, finances, and family problems, which lead to a fatigued feeling during the daytime.

Dealing with Your Anger

At some point after the shock of your rheumatic disease diagnosis finally sinks in, there may be a period of time where you experience significant anger. You may even feel some anger towards yourself. You may wrongly blame yourself for the presence of your condition, reasoning usually incorrectly that perhaps if you had taken better care of yourself that this might have been avoided. You also may be angry at yourself for not trying to help yourself more, especially if you are not doing enough to take back control of your arthritis. In most cases, of course, you personally had nothing to do with the onset of your rheumatic disease. Genetics, factors related to your immune system, and just the element of chance alone had much more to do with it. Unfortunately, most people try to assign blame for their situation. Some patients are just plain angry about the condition itself. They detest the "roller-coaster" ups and downs of their disease. They can't stand the constant fatigue or the predicament of never really feeling well. Patients are frustrated with their functional limitations and the impact that this is having on their daily lives at home and at work. Some patients feel significant anger towards a spouse or their children. This is particularly a problem if family members do not empathize and do not provide adequate support for the arthritic sufferer. When your disease flares up you may need and expect a helping hand from your family. This is "payback" after having provided for them over the years. You might expect that they would jump at the opportunity to reciprocate, especially at this time of need. It is extraordinarily disappointing when this does not happen.

You may also feel guilty or embarrassed for experiencing some feelings of anger toward God for putting you through all of this. Why has He singled out you to experience all of this suffering? Did you do something personally to trigger this lifelong "punishment"? If there are things in your life for which you are ashamed, then you may feel guilty and blame your disease on mistakes that you committed in years past.

You may be angry about work-related issues. You may be upset that you cannot do your job well. If you cannot fulfill your work requirements, you may be angry about the repercussions of your work limitations. You may be unable to improve your position and salary at your job. You also may be angry and feel trapped because you realize that if you do not remain gainfully employed, there will be financial consequences. You then might be unable to afford your medications. You also could potentially lose your medical insurance, which might be a disaster for you. Also, if you can't work due to your condition, you may severely disappoint your spouse as well as your family members. The financial consequences may have a great impact on their lives. Also if you don't show up for work periodically due to flare-ups in your condition, you may feel that you are disappointing other workers and simultaneously increasing their workload.

Whether or not you have job-related issues, you still may be angry about all the financial cost associated with your arthritis. Arthritis can put a severe dent in your pocketbook. Medication expenses add up quickly, especially if you have an aggressive form of inflammatory arthritis which may necessitate use of the newer biologic therapies. There may be costs related to doctor visits or hospitalizations. You may need to purchase aids to help you deal with activities of daily living, such as a wheelchair or motorized scooter, and these certainly are not cheap. As these costs add up, so does your resentment about having your rheumatic condition. When you can't afford to go out to a nice restaurant or take a vacation because of your medication costs, of course you are going to be angry about it. For some of you it is much worse than this, in that you are having to choose between your disease-related costs and putting food on the table, or buying clothes for yourself or your family. This is a most frustrating and demoralizing situation to have to face on a daily basis.

These are just some of the reasons that arthritis patients feel anger. If you are going to successfully take back control of your arthritis, you need to address these feelings. Anger can tear away at your insides and can be extremely self-destructive. Anger can add to feelings of stress and anxiety. These conditions can interfere with the ability of your immune system to function effectively. Your anger, therefore, can actually interfere with your ability to get well, especially if you need the help of your immune system to respond and help control your condition. It is important for you to do a better job of recognizing that you are angry. You need to identify the sources of your anger and deal with them. You may need to spend time having open and frank discussions with your family members. You certainly should discuss your feelings with your physician. He or she may be able to clarify whether any of your feelings of anger are justified. Perhaps if there is more of an explanation from your doctor about the nature and underlying causes of your condition, you will understand it better and stop blaming yourself for its development. You may need to spend more time dealing with your priest, minister, rabbi, or any other member of the clergy, and devote more time to prayer to resolve any anger you feel towards your Maker. It also may be extremely helpful to sit down with your boss at work and explain your situation and your medical problems. Let everyone at work know that in your heart of hearts you really want to do a terrific job. When your disease has quieted down, you can demonstrate this to them by being an exemplary employee and doing as much as you can to assist your employer and co-workers. Then when you have a flare-up, they may be much more willing to "dig in" and cover for you.

Therefore, by confronting the sources of your anger one by one and dealing with them in an open and effective way, you may be able to gradually reduce and eventually eliminate these very detrimental feelings. Once you do, you will be less impeded from taking back more control of your arthritis.

Dealing with Your Anxiety

Besides the anger that the rheumatic disease patient feels, there often is a heightened degree of anxiety in a number of areas. Many people are anxious about just going to see a doctor, let alone having fears associated with getting blood drawn or receiving an injection in a joint or muscle. You may feel anxious about the potential side effects that might occur with your various medications. Some therapies can theoretically harm important organs, and this has to be of some concern to you. As noted previously, the cost of these treatments also adds to your anxiety about your finances and whether you will be able to make ends meet. You worry that if you cannot work, your insurance coverage may lapse and then you will really be in financial hot water. Depending on how solid your relationship is with your "significant other," you may feel some anxiety about whether that person might walk out on you because of your illness. Perhaps he or she does not cope well with sickness and cannot handle the extra burdens imposed on them by your condition. You also have to deal with the general anxieties that involve all of the unknown factors related to your illness. Will your disease leave you disabled? Will it shorten your lifespan? Will it affect your cognitive functions? These are just but a few of the questions that are plaguing you. When you first are diagnosed with rheumatic illness, all of these myriad worries seem to run together. No wonder you feel anxious! In order to take back control of your anxiety, you need to first recognize that you are feeling anxious. Sometimes anxiety may be associated with sweaty palms, a rapid heart rate, breathlessness, sleeping problems, or feelings of "panic." To allay your anxiety, you need to address each of your concerns with your doctor and family members. Your physician will be able to counsel you regarding your disease and your prognosis and properly address each of your fears. If you follow the 12 critical steps described in this book, this will provide you with an excellent strategy to re-gain control of your arthritis. The 12 step approach gives you a sense of structure, and this foundation will help you to overcome much of the anxiety that you are feeling.

Why Bad Arthritis Happens to Good People

One of the most difficult dilemmas for a person who has religious convictions and claims to believe in God is dealing with the existence of evil in the world. Rabbi Kushner, in his classic best selling book on this subject, dealt with the issue of why bad things happen to good people. Throughout history horrible, catastrophic events have caused people repeatedly to question the existence of God after these events have taken place. This was certainly true among Jews all over the world after the Holocaust. How could God allow something like this to happen if he truly exists?

These same questions arose after the September 11 terrorist attack on the World Trade Center. How could God allow so many innocent people to die in this manner? I remember listening to Rabbi Kushner speak on television after these attacks. He pointed out that God was certainly not present in the evil terrorists who were involved in these dastardly acts. Instead, God was present in the acts of courage by the policemen, firemen, and emergency workers rendering care and risking their lives for others. God imbued the spirits of those who came forward to help others in need.

In applying this to rheumatic disease, God is not in the deformity and destruction that may be taking place in the joints. God is not in the morning stiffness or the fatigue that you may feel. If you look around you, however, you may see that God is in the love and support that you receive from your spouse and family members. God may be revealed in the care and sympathy that you receive from a very understanding and devoted physician, and members of the physician's staff. God may be working through neighbors who lend you a helping hand or from fellow members of a support group. Your rheumatologic condition will certainly act as a true test of your faith. Some of you may see this as an ultimate challenge. Those people who seem to do the best at dealing with their medical problems are the ones who find God in everyone around them and who stop blaming God for their predicament. None of us has the omniscience to understand how God truly works and why God does the things that He does in the universe. We have relatively small minds that can't possibly comprehend some divine master plan. If you truly want to get well, you need to deal with any "issues" that you have and re-establish your faith and trust in a Higher Being.

Don't Become the Person Who Family and Friends Avoid

In trying to take back control of your arthritis as well as your emotional state, it is important to spend some time looking into the mirror and assessing how other people may perceive you. If you are the kind of person who constantly complains about your predicament, then you will find that some members of your family along with friends and acquaintances will tend to avoid you. Many individuals find it burdensome to listen to your troubles. They have difficulty enough coping with their own set of problems. Their way of coping with your predicament is to avoid you altogether. If you are the kind of person that frequently tends to impose on family and friends, then once again many of them may gradually stop calling you. Not surprisingly they will eventually stop returning your phone messages. You may have requested help from them with shopping, transportation (including your medical visits) or even financial matters. Money issues probably drive away friends and family the quickest.

If your rheumatic disease has contributed to a state of depression, you may become "a real downer" to be around. If people always feel depressed when they spend any time with you, their solution may be to avoid doing so in the future. Therefore, it is important to take a good look at your behavior. Some of you may feel particularly trapped by your disease. You feel that you must call on family and friends to help you because you have no other alternative. If you are forced to do this, you should certainly express to them how extremely grateful you are for their help. Try to be as upbeat as possible when you are with these very supportive individuals. Even if at times you are "play-acting," this will help avoid your being isolated by everyone because you make them feel sad when they are with you. Many of you are aware of this and sensitized to these issues. In fact, some of you go overboard not to ask for help even when you need it. Often, family members complain that, "Mother doesn't allow us to give her the assistance that she needs." When you avoid calling on your family completely, this can be going too far in the opposite direction. Certainly, you should allow your family and friends to help you deal with your medical problems. Try to strike the proper balance between accepting their love and support for you and not "dragging them down" or overimposing on them.

Become an Inspiration for Others

Rather than depressing other people with a negative attitude, you instead have the unique opportunity to use your medical condition to actually inspire your family and friends. All of these individuals are most likely fully aware of the pain and suffering that you have to contend with on a daily basis. If you demonstrate a strong will not to give in to the arthritis and the pain and a desire to overcome it, others around you will be inspired by your courage. By setting an example for others with your will to live and commitment to conquer your condition, you will motivate others to fight against their own physical and emotional problems. If you can maintain a positive outlook and keep a smile on your face, you can have a tremendous influence on everyone in your life. You will have the capacity to turn the devastation of your illness into a positive example for others. This is one of the ultimate ways that you can truly take back control of your arthritis—by conquering your arthritis in an unbelievably courageous manner and thereby altering your destiny and the meaning and significance of your life.

Being Depressed for Good Reason

Clinical studies have shown that a vast majority of individuals with significant rheumatic diseases experience depression at some point during the course of their illness. In many cases, there is good reason to be upset or depressed. Just being in constant pain can contribute to feelings of depression. The possibility that you might lose some of your physical abilities can certainly "get you down." The impact that this may have on your ability to earn a living for your family or compete effectively in the workplace may weigh heavily upon you. You may be depressed over not being able to fulfill your responsibilities and role in the home. Men have feelings of inadequacy when they cannot do repairs around the house or handle heavy yard work. Women who work as home managers may fall behind with their household chores and may be disturbed by their inability to keep the home in immaculate shape. The fatigue that is often associated with rheumatic conditions may interfere with your ability to do a good job as a parent. You may not have the energy to attend all of your children's activities as you had done prior to your illness. This may result in your thinking that you are letting your children down. This in turn may make you feel sad and guilty. The added expense of your illness and the cost of medications may be putting an extra strain on the family's finances and these mounting financial worries can lead to depressed feelings as well.

Therefore, there are a large number of reasons why it is appropriate for arthritis patients to feel depressed. They are simply assessing their predicament and its impact on the home, workplace, finances, and their physical condition, and they are saddened by what they see. If this lasts for less than several months, and the individual learns to deal more effectively with these issues, then this is considered appropriate behavior. If, however, these feelings continue on for a longer time span, then the depression may take on "a life of its own" and become a separate medical problem that needs to be addressed and treated.

Just Plain Depressed

If you find yourself feeling sad and "blue" for a prolonged period of time, you may actually be experiencing full-blown depression. Most individuals tend to deny this at first and delude themselves into thinking that they are handling things effectively on their own. Family and friends may have a better vantage point and may realize that your depressed feelings are more significant long before you are able to arrive at the same conclusion. What are the clues and clinical symptoms that can help you to examine your own situation and determine whether you truly have depression?

Depression is not only a prolonged feeling of sadness, but also may be manifested by an increased degree of hyperirritability. You may become extremely quick-tempered and find yourself snapping at your spouse or your children, or having a "short fuse" at work.

Some individuals who are depressed find that they no longer enjoy the same things that previously made them happy. They may stop going out socially or stop participating in physical activities that were previously an important and integral part of their lives. Depression, therefore, leads to a diminished interest in things that were formerly pleasurable.

A person's appetite can actually change with the onset of depression. There can be either a marked decrease or a significant increase in appetite. People who lose their appetites will watch their weight drop off considerably, while others will find themselves constantly going to the refrigerator and overeating with a resultant increase in weight.

With depression, there may be a change in one's sleep pattern. Some depressed individuals may sleep much of the time, even during daytime hours. Others will have the opposite problem with insomnia and a lack of restful sleep.

Sometimes with depression there can be a severe lack of sufficient energy to perform physical activities. These individuals often find themselves just sitting around much of the time. Others may have an opposite response where they feel quite fidgety and restless.

One of the more common manifestations of depression is a feeling of worthlessness with a marked decrease in one's self-esteem. You may find yourself feeling guilty about past events or mistakes you have made throughout your life. These seem to rise to the surface and weigh heavily upon you with the onset of your depression.

Sometimes depressed people will find they have a great deal of difficulty concentrating. It is sometimes hard to think clearly or focus thoughts properly. Some people will have problems with their recollection of facts and figures. These problems can particularly affect job performance, especially if your work requires sharp and clear thinking.

Depressed individuals will often feel fatigued with a marked loss of energy. If you are depressed you may feel that you are just dragging about much of the time without the "get up and go" to participate in any type of a meaningful exercise program.

Finally, the most worrisome symptoms of depression are persistent thoughts of death or committing suicide. A severely depressed person may be suffering from profound feelings of hopelessness and despair.

If a number of these symptoms apply to your own situation, you may be considered clinically depressed. Instead of continuing to deny your state of depression, you should bring these symptoms to the attention of your physician so that he or she is aware of them.

If you are going to make a genuine effort to take back control of your arthritis, you will need to get treatment for any associated depression in addition to the therapy directed at your underlying rheumatic disease. The good news is that there are excellent new treatments now available with far fewer side effects than traditional anti-depressants upon which we used to rely. Although medications such as Elavil (amitriptyline) and Pamelor (nortriptyline) are effective, they occasionally cause side effects. They have largely given way to a new category of antidepressants called serotonin re-uptake inhibitors (SSRIs). This group includes Prozac (fluoxetine), Zoloft (sertraline), Paxil (paroxetine), Celexa (citalopram), and Lexapro (escitalopram). Far more patients are able to tolerate these drugs with successful improvement of their depression. This has helped lift them out of the depths of despair and correct many of the symptoms delineated above. Once depression is better controlled, patients with rheumatic diseases are then able to participate in physical activities including a formal exercise program. The endorphins released in the brain as a result of this exercise will then help improve the patient's depression in a more natural way. It is possible that over time and by following the 12 critical steps to take back control of your arthritis, the improvement in your physical condition will help lead to a resolution of these depressed feelings.

Stop Denying Your Condition and Learn to Accept It

A great many patients will experience symptoms for a number of months before finally making an appointment to see a physician to find out if they truly have arthritis or not. This is often due to the fact that many people go through a period of denial, refusing to accept the fact that they might be ill.

Many patients are reluctant to make necessary changes in their daily habits or work patterns even after being informed of their diagnosis. I tend to see this type of behavior more often in male patients than in female arthritic patients. "Macho" working-age men have a particularly tough time dealing with their inability to continue to perform manual labor. Some patients diagnosed with active inflammatory arthritis, such as rheumatoid arthritis, will continue to perform detrimental activities at work. This is in spite of knowing that this is likely to trigger further pain, swelling, and joint damage. Men and women are guilty of denial when it comes to chores around the house. Male patients with severe arthritis come to their office visits and tell me about increased joint pain after digging post holes for a new fence or after trimming trees or repairing the roof. Women who should know better are out in the yard lifting or moving heavy flowerpots or digging and weeding. Patients need to move beyond their denial to learn to be more accepting of their medical situations.

If you are in a state of denial and are having trouble accepting your diagnosis, you will not be psychologically ready to follow all 12 critical steps to take back control of your arthritis. You first need to come to grips with your condition and understand what is likely to happen to you if you do not follow these steps and continue to ignore your doctor's advice. Once you get over the initial "shock" of your diagnosis, you can move on to a more productive phase called "acceptance," where you can begin to map out an effective strategy for fighting back. With the help of loved ones, other arthritis patients, your physician and up-to-date arthritis information, you can start doing everything in your power to fight against your rheumatic disease and maximize your outcome. With a positive outlook and an acceptance of your rheumatic condition, you can then start out on the challenging path to take back control of your arthritis.

The Power of Prayer

Twenty years ago, most physicians might have been reluctant to talk to their patients about using prayer as an important aspect of treatment for their rheumatic condition. Results from recent research, however, reinforced the huge potential benefits of prayer. The type of praying that most people are familiar with is petitionary prayer, which involves asking (petitioning) God to help you with your medical problems. A different type of prayer is intercessory prayer, with prayer by an individual or a group of people on behalf of others whom they know or don't know at all. The idea of praying for a list of total strangers to improve their disease outcome is still very controversial, but deserving of further study based on preliminary results.

It is not clear why prayer may be so helpful to patients. In the case of the rheumatic diseases, prayer may lead to a feeling of peace and inner tranquility that can result in an improved immune system. Prior research has shown changes occurring in the circulation to the brain during prayer or meditation. Prayer, therefore, has the capacity to produce physiologic changes in the body, including improved blood pressure and a more controlled pulse rate. Praying and meditating can significantly reduce feelings of anxiety. Prayer can also reduce feelings of depression. Thus, prayer can have an ameliorative effect on your rheumatic condition itself, the associated pain and suffering, and your attitude towards your disease. Prayer and meditation, therefore, should be yet another way to take back control of your arthritis.

Although the exact origins of the Serenity Prayer are unclear, it is still very applicable to arthritis patients. It may have been written by Dr. Niebuhr of the Union Theological Seminary, but other sources suggest that it may have been composed centuries earlier. The prayer has been associated with the Alcoholics Anonymous movement, but still is a good one for rheumatic disease patients to use as well. "God, grant me the serenity to accept things I cannot change, courage to change the things I can, and wisdom to know the difference."

Key Points in Taking Back Control of Your Emotions:

1. Pinpoint and address all of the reasons for feeling angry about your condition.

2. Discuss all of your fears and the sources of your anxious feelings with your doctor.

3. Reconcile with God and realize that you cannot possibly understand how God works.

4. Try to avoid being a real "downer" to be around.

5. Inspire others with the courage you show in handling your own rheumatic disorder.

6. Learn the difference between being appropriately depressed and experiencing depression as a separate condition.

7. Recognize the symptoms of depression and see if these apply to your situation.

8. Stop using denial to avoid dealing with your problems and learn to accept the reality of your medical condition.

9. Use the power of prayer as an important and integral part of your treatment program.

Step 11: Take Back Control of Your Sex Life

Telltale Signs That Your Sex Life Is in Trouble:

- Your spouse rarely hugs or kisses you in a loving way.

- Your spouse always comes home late and long after you are asleep and certainly too late to have sex.

- Your last orgasm occurred around the time that the Brooklyn Dodgers moved to Los Angeles.

- You feel embarrassed when you attempt to pleasure yourself by masturbating.

- You have trouble getting aroused when you or your partner touch your private parts.

- Your pain during intercourse prevents you from climaxing.

- You have vaginal pain with intercourse due to severe dryness.

- You are constantly aware of your arthritic pain throughout your attempt at sexual activity.

- You never discuss your sexual desires and needs with your partner.

- Your pain medication makes you feel too sleepy to consider trying or enjoying sex.

- You are depressed and don't feel at all desirable and cannot understand why anyone would even think of having sex with you, even if you were the last person on earth.

The Impact of Arthritis on Your Sex Life

One of the greatest pleasures in life is having sex and experiencing the ecstasy of an orgasm. Unfortunately, in patients with musculo-skeletal problems, sexual pleasure may be difficult to achieve due to the physical as well as psychological factors that are associated with these conditions. In the last chapter, I discussed emotional aspects of having a disease that may be deforming and disabling. Depression and anxiety certainly play a role in your ability or inability to enjoy sex and be able to fully climax.

Patients with rheumatic diseases often have low self-esteem, which comes after they start realizing that they are no longer as physically capable as they were when they were healthy. Household chores now are more difficult to accomplish. Holding down gainful employment to support oneself and one's family may no longer be in the cards. As your joints begin to show deformities, you no longer feel physically attractive. You may have difficulty looking at your own joints, let alone wanting others to see you in this shape. If you are on medications, there may be undesirable physical side effects. Corticosteroids may cause significant weight gain and facial swelling (mooned facies), which markedly changes your appearance. Traditional NSAIDs or aspirin can cause unsightly bruising over your limbs (ecchymoses). Certain medications like methotrexate or Arava (leflunomide) may result in significant hair loss. Thus, your self-image may be severely damaged by one or more of these factors.

A substantial number of patients with rheumatic diseases will, therefore, feel lonely and isolated. Any acts of repulsion or rejection by your partner will just reinforce your own self-doubt and validate your feelings of worthlessness. You actually harbor an even greater need for acceptance and love than a normal healthy individual. You have a deep need to be held and caressed and given expressions of love and commitment. You need your spouse to recognize and acknowledge that it is still the same soul present within you that he/she loves, even if your outward appearance has been changed. This acceptance by your partner of who you truly are, and the lesser importance of the "physical you" is most important in being able to cope with the ravages of many of these diseases.

Physical Limitations That Interfere with Sexual Activity

There is no question that arthritis and its subsequent physical limitations may potentially interfere with "traditional" forms of sexual activity. The most common sexual position used in having intercourse, the so-called "missionary position," requires that the male partner be able to at least temporarily support a portion of his own body weight on his wrists and shoulders. If there is active inflammation in these joints, it may be too painful to continue in this position. The woman with hip joint involvement will have difficulty in allowing the hips to fall outwardly (abduction of the hips) to permit her male partner to enter her. Your hands are very much needed and involved throughout sexual activity. You certainly use your hands a great deal as part of foreplay in fondling your partner. Your hands are necessary to pleasure yourself by masturbating. Thus, involvement of the joints of the hands with arthritis can make sex more difficult. Other individuals may experience involvement of the tempero-mandibular joint of the jaw as part of their arthritis. If this occurs in a female, it may then be extremely painful to have oral sex and perform fellatio.

Pain Can Decrease Sexual Pleasure

Not only is joint pain limiting in terms of the actual sexual act itself, but the pain may be severe enough that it interferes with your sexual desire (libido). It is really hard to concentrate on your genitalia when your brain is constantly being bombarded with painful impulses coming back from one or more joints. This creates an enormous conflict between painful and pleasurable signals. As I will discuss below, there are ways to ensure that the painful impulses are suppressed enough so that the pleasurable stimuli can win out.

When you have arthritis, you may have fears or anticipation that the pain is about to return or worsen. Experience has also taught you that if you engage in any strenuous physical activity this may aggravate your pain or hasten its return. Thus, participating in any very physical sexual activity may bring on the pain. There will be some concern that this could happen at any moment in the midst of the heat of passion, and this could interfere with your ability to permit yourself to enjoy sex. It also could impair your capacity to reach climax. You may be satisfied by just pleasuring your partner and not prolonging things in order for you to have an orgasm. In your mind, you are more concerned that you will aggravate your joints at some point if you try to stretch your luck. This may create enough mental tension that you will find it impossible to relax while having sex. Even a healthy person knows that if he/she is extremely tense or anxious that it will be virtually impossible to experience an orgasm. If you combine the ever-present pain along with emotional factors that are working against the arthritis sufferer, you can understand why it is more difficult to enjoy sex and experience orgasms with these conditions.

Depression and Sexual Interest

Depression is often manifested by a lack of interest in things that you used to find pleasurable. Nowhere is this more applicable than when it comes to sex. Since the majority of patients with significant arthritis go through a period of depression at some point during the course of their disease, sexual disinterest is a common finding in patients with rheumatic diseases. Anti-depressant medications may help to alleviate some of the depressed feelings that come with these dramatic changes in your physical capacity. Unfortunately, many of these drugs interfere with your libido and may, therefore, negate the benefits of feeling less depressed while on these medicines.

Female Issues: Pain, Dryness, Ulcerations, and Infections

Some women will have symptoms of painful intercourse (dyspareunia), which may be secondary to dryness of the vaginal mucosa. This can be seen in postmenopausal females who have become estrogen deficient. Oral hormone replacement therapy or topical vaginal estrogen cream may be indicated in this situation. You would have to check with your gynecologist to determine if you lack normal vaginal secretions and to see if you are a candidate for any of these treatments. Recent reports regarding an increased risk of strokes or cancer of the breast or uterus with hormonal treatment have steered patients and physicians away from these medications. Therefore, the pros and cons of this type of therapy need to be fully discussed with your gynecologist.

Other women who have vaginal dryness and yet are not postmenopausal may have developed this as a result of having Sjogren's syndrome. In this rheumatic condition, patients experience an autoimmune assault by their own cells on the mucosal glands including the eyes, mouth, and vaginal areas. Patients come in to see the rheumatologist, gynecologist, ophthalmologist, or otolaryngologist (ENT) complaining about dryness in one or more of these areas. Sjogren's syndrome may occur on its own, but also may be seen in association with other rheumatic conditions such as systemic lupus erythematosus, scleroderma, or rheumatoid arthritis. Some patients who still have some capacity to make tears, saliva, or vaginal mucus may benefit from medications like pilocarpine (Salagen) or the more recently released cevimeline (Evoxac). If there is no residual activity remaining in the mucous glands, then these medications are unlikely to be of much benefit. Patients with vaginal dryness, whether secondary to Sjogren's syndrome or postmenopausal changes, will experience significantly less vaginal pain with the use of ample lubricants such as K-Y jelly or Vaseline Intensive Care lotion. Also saliva from your partner works as an excellent natural lubricant.

Another reason that a woman may have problems with intercourse is the formation of vaginal ulcerations. This may occur in systemic lupus erythematosus patients. Other patients may experience vaginal ulcers secondary to medication. This may be seen infrequently with methotrexate therapy, a treatment that is now a mainstay of therapy in rheumatoid arthritis as well as psoriatic arthritis. The concurrent use of folic acid is intended to prevent mucosal ulcerations, but it is not always one hundred per cent effective in doing so.

Some women may avoid sexual intercourse due to vaginal fungal infections with monilia. This is commonly seen in patients who are taking higher doses of steroids that may be required to treat systemic forms of vasculitis or active forms of lupus. It also may be seen in patients who are on immunosuppressive drugs that may be needed for the treatment of lupus nephritis (kidney involvement) or lupus cerebritis (central nervous system involvement of the brain). There may be a thick "cheesy" type of whitish discharge from the vagina associated with vaginal irritation. Your gynecologist may be able to eradicate this with the use of oral medications, vaginal anti-fungal suppositories and cream. Your rheumatologist, of course, should make every effort to reduce your corticosteroid or immunosuppressive medication level, if possible, in order to avoid chronic or recurrent problems.

Other medications may cause some additional problems. Many patients are taking pain medicines (analgesics) to try to control the pain from their arthritis. The stronger drugs are narcotics and may have a sedating effect on you. It is hard to be able to participate in sexual activity and even harder to experience an orgasm if you are extremely sleepy and lacking much energy.

What Your Partner May Be Thinking and Feeling

The entire problem with pleasurable sex does not only focus on the arthritis sufferer. Your partner's thoughts, feelings, and fears also play a role. Oftentimes, a healthy person holds back on having very physical or passionate sex because they are afraid that they might somehow injure their partner. At the very least, they worry about just causing their loved one a higher degree of pain following such intense physical exertion.

If this has happened previously, then he/she will feel guilty even bringing up the subject of sexual activity based on past experiences. The healthy partner will feel that they are being extremely selfish in asking that the arthritis sufferer help pleasure them when they know that their partner is in pain. If you have a healthy spouse who has been avoiding sexual activity, you might have misinterpreted their behavior as a lack of interest and caring, as opposed to being related to a genuine concern about not making matters worse for you.

The Impact of Arthritis on Different Sexual Relationships

I would like for you to consider several different scenarios. First think about the situation where the male is the one with arthritis and the woman is healthy. When she first met you and you were healthy, you may have fulfilled her desires of marrying a strong virile individual who would be her protector. She wanted a person who could provide for her and be her breadwinner. Now that your body has been changed significantly as a result of your arthritis, and you no longer can be gainfully employed, you find yourself having to deal with your own feelings of inadequacy and low self-worth. On the other hand, she has to deal with all of her feelings of disappointment along with additional worries about her finances and her own future because of your illness. These feelings will certainly need to be dealt with if you are going to be able to make love with one another successfully.

In the second scenario, contemplate the situation where the woman has arthritis and the male is healthy. The man is disappointed because he can no longer have the spontaneous, wild, and passionate sex that he desires. He also may be upset by the fact that he is now called upon to perform a lot of the household chores that his wife used to handle. The woman not only has to deal with all of her own pain and suffering, but now she has to worry whether her man might start to stray and look for other sexual outlets.

In the final scenario, think of a situation where both people have arthritis. Life, of course, may be harder for both of you when there is not at least one healthy partner to take care of the heavier types of activities that need to be done. Sex may be even more challenging for both of you in trying to get things coordinated when both individuals have their own separate physical issues. From a psychological aspect, however, it may be an easier situation to deal with since both of you understand what it is truly like to be afflicted by arthritis and can totally empathize with one another.

Failed Marriages Due to Arthritis

Not surprisingly there is a significant rate of divorce once one partner in a marriage develops arthritis. When the healthy partner leaves, it may be because that individual is incapable of dealing with illness involving someone close to them. In some cases, there may have been some problems in the marriage from the start. The subsequent development of a rheumatic illness becomes the proverbial "straw that broke the camel's back." There may be additional financial pressures created when one of the salaries that you both were counting on now is lost. Certainly, there may be additional costs related to the expense of doctor visits, hospitalizations, diagnostic tests, and medications. You may be forced to choose between buying your medications or being able to afford a nice dinner out or taking in a movie. Resentment may, therefore, build up as your disease saps your financial reserves.

Recall the second scenario that I described where the man was healthy, but the wife had arthritis. He may not be too thrilled about being "domesticated" and having to wash the clothes and dishes. For some men, this role reversal challenges their very masculinity. In a "me-first" era like we are currently experiencing, it may be very difficult for a man to be so self-sacrificing and put his own needs secondary to the needs of his ill wife. This is part of the reason that frequently when the going gets tough, some of the tough guys get going and fly the coop. As I stated earlier, if there are cracks already forming in the relationship, then the additional strains associated with the onset of a debilitating and incapacitating illness may cause the cracks to expand into a huge abyss and threaten to permanently and irrevocably wreck your marriage. On the other hand, if you are lucky enough to have married a most loving and supportive spouse, then there will never be anything in life that will tear you apart. An arthritic illness will be seen by both of you as just another one of life's challenges that you need to conquer together. With this type of loving relationship, taking back control of your sex life, which has been spoiled by your arthritic problems, is readily doable with the helpful tips I will delineate for you.

The Benefits of Pleasurable Sex in the Arthritis Patient

There are significant potential benefits for the arthritis patient who is able to learn successful techniques to achieve pleasurable sex, in spite of his or her condition. Having good and regular sex will serve to boost your self-esteem and self-worth. It will lift up your self-confidence. When you have an orgasm, the brain releases chemicals called endorphins, and these are natural painkillers. Thus, after you finish climaxing you may experience less pain than before you started. This is certainly an added bonus for any arthritis sufferer.

Good Communication Leads to Better Sex

The first important step then, in taking back control of your sex life, is to establish open communications with your partner so that misinterpretations and misunderstandings do not occur. Rather than keeping your true feelings and needs hidden from your partner, a patient with arthritis has to learn how to candidly discuss all aspects of their sexual activity. For some, who are more romantically inclined and prefer spontaneity, this may be hard to accept and difficult to carry out, but it is essential. A whole host of items need to be clarified including the preferred times for sex, the most enjoyable positions, learning what feels particularly good and what hurts, discussing what foreplay works the best, as well as talking about many other concerns. One very important thing to agree upon is a specific signal that can be used at any time during sex to indicate that the other partner needs to stop whatever they are doing because it is painful. It might be that two taps on the skin means to stop and try something different or to pause and find out what you are doing that is increasing your partner's discomfort level. That way you can also be made aware not to repeat the same activity in the future.

Sexual Timing is Important

Arthritis patients have already discovered over the years what time of the day they feel the best. Rheumatoid arthritis patients, in general, have their worst time in the morning due to the profound morning stiffness that they may experience. While the patient has been sleeping, microscopic strands have formed within the inflamed joints. It usually takes an hour or more to break these up following a nice hot shower and by gradually working the joints through their range of motion. Thus, sex at sunrise for a rheumatoid arthritis patient would usually be the worst time to choose. On the other hand, later in the day, after the stiffness has disappeared and the medicines have kicked in, would be a considerably better time to have sex.

Osteoarthritis patients do not experience much morning stiffness (usually less than fifteen to thirty minutes), but they tend to have more pain towards the end of the day after using their degenerated joints throughout the day. For them, having sex within one to two hours of arising might be preferred.

If a person afflicted with arthritis is working full time, then by the time he/she arrives home at night exhaustion may already have set in. It might be prudent to forget about having sex during the workweek, but instead try to get together on the weekend when both of you are more rested. Also on

Saturday and Sunday there will be significantly more time to allow for proper preparation and foreplay and for the sexual acts themselves. So, as you can see, timing is an important consideration.

Timing your medicines correctly may also make sex much more pleasurable. It is best to try to take your pain medicines about twenty to thirty minutes before you start making love. Hopefully, their beneficial effect will then kick in precisely when you need it most. You need to figure out how much medicine you can comfortably take without getting overly sleepy, which could, in turn, interfere with your sexual capability.

Your NSAID dose could also be similarly timed to be taken thirty to sixty minutes before any sexual activity to take advantage of the analgesic effect it provides you. If you have a lot of muscular tightness or spasm as part of your condition, a muscle relaxant might be taken thirty minutes prior to sex to help relax you and your muscles. Obviously if you are overly relaxed, you may not be able to perform. This is similar to the negative effect of too much sedating pain medicine.

Forget About Spontaneity for Greater Sexual Enjoyment

I hope that I have made it clear to you that sex for an arthritis sufferer is usually a planned activity. Spontaneous sex might actually be detrimental for you. If your muscles are tight and you have not done all of the preliminary things that I am suggesting, then you could easily strain one of your muscles. You may then wind up with an injury from your sudden passionate physical activity. Having agreed with your partner on a specific time, you should start your preparation for sex with a warm shower or hot tub bath. Your partner may even choose to join you! You already have taken your medications at precisely the right time to give you maximal benefit.

Following this, a gentle massage of your muscles by your partner will help loosen you up. At the same time, your relaxing hot tub bath and massage are definitely getting you into the right frame of mind. The fact that your spouse is being so tender and loving to you all the while, and making you feel so good, is instilling in you a desire to return the favor and give true pleasure back. You may want to even add some nice limbering and stretching exercises after your shower or bath that may lessen any discomfort and decrease the chance of an injury with your upcoming physical activity.

Now You Are Ready to Rock and Roll

Now that you are warmed up, you may commence your lovemaking. Things should start off slowly with a great deal of gentle fondling, caressing, and kissing. Take your time so that you both can derive the greatest pleasure out of this intimate time together.

You may want to start off with some oral sexual activity. For the arthritis male individual whose wife gives him fellatio, not only will this feel great and prepare him for intercourse, but it also may give him confirmation of her love and appreciation of him. For the female rheumatic disease patient, oral sex will help lubricate the vaginal tissues and make penetration by the healthy partner less painful. You can also use the topical lotions and lubricants that I mentioned earlier.

In the discussions with your partner that are essential to maximize your chances of having pleasurable sex, you should have already established what feels good and what hurts. Painful activities should be strictly taboo, even if the other person happens to particularly enjoy it. There are so many other ways to safely pleasure one another that alternative techniques need to be explored and perfected.

Getting Creative

When you were both healthy, you might never have felt compelled to add sex toys to your lovemaking. These various "devices," however, may be particularly "user-friendly" to the arthritis patient. Vibrators and dildos for females, such as the popular Pocket Rocket and the even more highly touted Rabbit will help you to successfully masturbate and may also be used in conjunction with having intercourse. There are other specific massage devices that may be used on men. The Internet has now made these sex shops accessible to everyone with a computer. It is no longer necessary to drive down to the local sex shop in sunglasses and a trench coat to avoid being recognized when making such purchases.

As part of all of this foreplay, you may also want to watch a sexually explicit movie to arouse you, or flip through a sex magazine together. Most cable and satellite companies offer Playboy as a special channel, and this may help get you both more aroused.

Alternative Sexual Positions

There are a number of alternatives to the missionary position that might be easier for you. With both individuals lying on their side and the man situated behind the woman, the man can attempt to enter the woman's vagina from behind. This position avoids stressing the woman's hips, and avoids putting too much pressure on the man's upper extremity joints. Another alternative is for both of you to be in the standing position with the woman leaning on some type of elevated surface (this may be a table-top with a couple of large pillows on it). The man then enters the vagina from a rear approach with the woman bent slightly forward. Whatever position you use, make sure that both individuals are comfortable and pain free so that you both can enjoy having intercourse together.

Sex in Spite of Flare-Ups in Your Arthritis

It should be expected that there will be times when your sexual activity will have to be modified due to flare-ups in your arthritis. You may even choose to hold off on things until new or higher doses of medicine kick in and get your condition under better control. You may need to rely more on manual manipulation or oral sex by your partner during these more difficult periods. Of course, you always can utilize masturbation if having intercourse is out of the question. You, more than anyone else, know exactly what feels good and how to pleasure yourself without causing additional pain.

Have Fun

So now that you have familiarized yourself with these considerations regarding sexual activity in spite of having arthritis, you should be ready to take back control of your sex life. Remember that sex is supposed to be fun and enjoyable! At first, when you start to institute many of these suggestions, you may feel like it is too controlled and planned, and less spontaneous than you might prefer. Once you have all of the ground rules worked out, however, it eventually will start to feel more natural to you. In the end, both you and your partner will be more anxious to have sex, knowing that you will be receiving great pleasure from one another.

Key Points in Taking Back Control of Your Sex Life:

1. Open up channels of communications about your sexual likes and dislikes.

2. Time the taking of your NSAIDs, pain pills, or muscle relaxants to give you the maximum benefit during your sexual activity.

3. Pick the optimal time of the day and the best days of the week to have sex.

4. In preparation for sex, include a hot tub bath or shower, muscle stretching, and massage.

5. Include plenty of time for foreplay.

6. Agree with your partner about the most comfortable sexual positions for intercourse.

7. Be willing to be innovative and explore new sexual experiences, such as using sex toys and viewing stimulating and sexually explicit materials. Don't be embarrassed about including masturbation in your sexual repertoire.

8. Agree upon a signal that quickly indicates to your partner that you are experiencing more pain so that he/she can stop what they are doing and move on to something that is pleasurable.

9. If you are experiencing a flare-up of your disease, temporarily change over to manual techniques, oral sex, or masturbation until your illness is controlled well enough so that you can enjoy intercourse once again.

10. Remember that even with arthritis, sex can be fun and pleasurable. It can also increase your self-esteem while helping to release all of those soothing endorphins that may help to decrease your pain.

Step 12: Take Back Control of Your Information About Arthritis

Telltale Signs That You Are Not in Control of Your Arthritis Information Sources:

- You do not understand the medical terms the doctor uses at your visits.

- You do not understand why various tests are being done on you and what the abnormal results mean.

- You do not have an understanding of your medications, how they work, and what side effects to expect.

- You are not familiar with the newer revolutionary treatments for arthritis.

- You have no contact with other patients who have a similar medical condition and no one to communicate with who understands what you are going through.

- You do not know how to search the Internet in order to find additional medical information.

- You are not familiar with support groups in your local community dealing with your illness.

- You are not aware of books or video programs about arthritis or how to find out more information about these.

We Live in an Information Age

In the last decade we have experienced an astounding explosion of information on health related issues. With computers becoming faster and cheaper, more and more individuals have decided to participate in the computer age. Access to on-line information over the Internet affords the individual immediate updates on the latest research and treatments touching on virtually every health condition. Initially, there was some reluctance by our seniors to participate in this process. A large part of this was due to a lack of knowledge regarding the operation of a computer and dealing with the Worldwide Web. This portion of the population, however, has now become fully aware of the potential of these new technological advancements and people are logging on in greater numbers. The rheumatic diseases have not been left out of this new wave of information. There are web sites dedicated to all of the major specific rheumatic disorders as well as web sites focusing on the various medications that we use to treat the rheumatic diseases.

In addition to the Internet, there are numerous helpful books, which offer patients advice on how to cope with these conditions. Video programs are available at websites such as ArthritisMall.com, Amazon.com or through the Arthritis Foundation. The Arthritis Foundation provides pamphlets on every major rheumatic disease and specific treatments. An individual may obtain these free from their local Arthritis Foundation chapter. In major metropolitan areas in the United States, the Arthritis Foundation sponsors an Arthritis Information Day. This usually occurs during Arthritis Awareness Month in May of each year and features local rheumatologists speaking about different rheumatic diseases and their treatment. Thus if you use the Internet along with books, pamphlets, video programs, and community lectures, you will certainly have a sizeable amount of ancillary information to expand on what your rheumatologist has told you during your office visits.

Using the Internet to Your Advantage

If you are not already utilizing the Internet to help increase your knowledge about your medical conditions, then you need to find a way to do so. There are usually classes available in urban areas as part of adult education courses. You can check with your local public library, which usually provides Internet access free of charge. I would wager a guess that in most cases your children and grandchildren are totally computer literate and would probably relish the opportunity to share their knowledge with you. They can teach you how to navigate the Internet. I can't overemphasize the importance of your taking this critical step in order to place such an incredible amount of up-to-date information literally at your fingertips.

Warnings About the Information on the Internet

Those of you who have used the Internet for any length of time know that there is a wide variation in the reliability of the information provided. Just because something is in print on the Internet does not guarantee its truthfulness and accuracy. Written information on sites that are selling unproven remedies often contain glowing endorsements of the products for sale. Usually there are written testimonials included. All of this information is obviously designed to encourage you to purchase this particular product. The lay public may have trouble deciphering these types of websites versus legitimate ones.

There are some general rules of thumb, which may help you in trying to assess the validity of the information on a site. All of the medical pieces should be signed by a physician or licensed specialist in that particular area of expertise. It is helpful if there is some university affiliation of the writer or the website. It is less likely that a medical university with its strong sense of responsibility to the public would use its "good name" in some unethical manner. Also a physician who is affiliated with a major university medical center also would feel an obligation to the community to put out trustworthy information. An honor code logo may be displayed by those sites agreeing to adhere to a list of ethical standards, but this is not a one hundred per cent guarantee of the accuracy of the information presented on the site. Of course, you can certainly check out any information that you discover by bringing it to your own physician, especially if you have questions or doubts in your mind after visiting a particular site. Most physicians are aware that more and more of their patients are indeed searching the Internet.

Physicians who understand the importance of patient self-education should encourage their patients to utilize the Internet. If you have a physician who feels threatened by your efforts to enlighten yourself about your condition, then this should be troubling and might even tempt you to consider changing physicians.

One-Stop Shopping for Arthritis Information

When you search the Internet with the word "arthritis" you will find over six million responses. It is not likely that you will be willing to sort through even a portion of such a vast number of websites and references. Obviously, if you were able to go to one site that contained updated information on all of the basic rheumatic disorders as well as the latest therapies, this would make life a lot easier. When I was investigating various arthritis websites in 1999, I was flabbergasted at the lack of a website that guided the patient through all of the essential information to understand the diagnosis and treatment of arthritis and osteoporosis. Creating a comprehensive patient information site about arthritis was my motivation in developing the ArthritisCentral.com website. On this site you are provided with all of the basic tools an individual afflicted with arthritis would need to gain a basic understanding of arthritis. For example, instead of making you search for each new treatment for rheumatoid arthritis, all of these are discussed as Original Feature Articles on the site. When controversial issues are aired on television or in print, ArthritisCentral.com quickly tries to clarify these for you. For example, a recent television news report frightened Vioxx users with reports about a group of patients who developed meningitis. Within forty-eight hours there was a written article posted on ArthritisCentral.com clarifying the details of this story and reassuring Vioxx users. Hopefully ArthritisCentral.com was able to quickly put their minds at ease by informing patients that this was an extremely rare event. After physicians were alerted to news of a supply shortage of Enbrel, I investigated this situation further and then informed our ArthritisCentral.com visitors that this was not a problem related to unexpected side effects or any defect in the product. This was simply a production "snafu" that would be corrected in time. Once again, it was our hope at ArthritisCentral.com that our news story would spare Enbrel users unnecessary alarm based on the reports in the media.

Even though this book provides you with an excellent road map to deal with your arthritis, new information on the treatment of arthritis is constantly being published. ArthritisCentral.com can serve as your principal resource to keep up with the steady stream of new research and updates in therapy that you will need to be aware of in the coming months and years. Original Feature Articles at ArthritisCentral will summarize information on specific new medications including biologic response modifiers. Each week Arthritis Central subscribers receive a newsletter highlighting an important development in the diagnosis or treatment of rheumatic diseases. We also emphasize beneficial exercises designed for patients afflicted with arthritis.

Learning the Basics in Arthritis

If you are going to take back control of your arthritis, it is essential that you have a fundamental knowledge of arthritis.

This should include the terminology used, the differences among the most common types of arthritis (there are over one hundred rheumatic conditions), the various diagnostic tests available, and treatment options specific for each disorder. At ArthritisCentral.com we have gathered all of this information together for you at one location. The best way to start is to go to the Glossary of Terms and get familiar with the "lingo" used in dealing with rheumatic disorders. All of the major rheumatic conditions are presented in the form of interactive disease maps, which educate you regarding the symptoms, physical findings, laboratory and x-ray studies involved in making a correct diagnosis of a specific rheumatic disease. There is also information summarizing the treatment for each condition. There is an additional section with frequently asked questions about each of these major disorders as well. You then should move on to the tables displaying all of the laboratory and x-ray studies that might be performed in your case to ascertain a correct diagnosis. The tables indicate what an abnormal result is with an explanation of the significance of the test outcome. This may be extremely helpful to you in understanding why your doctor has ordered certain tests. It may also help you to better understand your results and their implication in your case. All of this general information is available free to anyone coming to the ArthritisCentral.com web site.

For those desiring a much broader range of information with more details on specific and newer forms of therapy, there is a subscriber portion of the site. It features Original Feature Articles on all of the newer therapies. This includes the newest anti-inflammatory medications including the selective COX-2 inhibitors (Celebrex, Vioxx and Bextra). There are special articles on the revolutionary biologic response modifiers (Enbrel, Humira, Remicade and Kineret). There are also original articles on all of the options for the treatment of osteoporosis including Fosamax, Actonel, Evista, Miacalcin nasal spray, and Forteo as well as promising treatments for the future. In each case, not only is information presented about the efficacy of these treatments, but also the reader is forewarned about key side effects that may occur with each of these.

The ArthritisCentral.com website is the home of Arthritis.TV, the largest collection of video programs on arthritis. One series of programs, called *Revolutionary Treatments for Arthritis*, highlights some of the newer biologic therapies now available for patients as well as other exciting and innovative treatments. Another series of programs is entitled *Arthritis Tonight: Stories of Courage, Persistence and Hope*. On these video programs, patients share with you their personal stories about arthritis and osteoporosis and how they have learned to overcome obstacles in order to get well. They point out insightful ways they have managed to deal with the pain and physical limitations from their arthritis. By listening to other patients, you, in turn, can learn to better cope with your own condition more effectively.

A third video series is called *Coping with Arthritis and Osteoporosis*. In this section are video programs on various exercise options. For example, we demonstrate ways to strengthen the hipbone in patients with osteoporosis. We have featured individual aquatic exercises for those afflicted with arthritis. One video shows you how to correctly utilize a cane when walking. In this section we have also included topics related to sexual issues confronting arthritis patients. We have presented video pieces on depression as well as on spiritual considerations in coping with these sometimes devastating illnesses.

A fifth series of programs includes our ArthritisCentral newscasts, which explain and clarify important up-to-date developments in the world of arthritis. Unlike the short sound bytes that you get on television, we are able to expand and explain in greater detail the relevance of each news event and the implications for you. Thus, the ArthritisCentral.com web site provides you with a tremendous starting point in the search for information and knowledge pertaining to the rheumatic diseases.

There are a number of additional outstanding general resources on the Internet that contain reliable information about the most common rheumatic disorders. In Appendix A, I have created a table that lists some of the best of these sites. There are also more specific websites that target specific rheumatic disorders. These are listed in a separate table in Appendix A.

Getting Your Family Involved

It is extremely important that you obtain as much information about your condition as possible from the many different sources that we have been discussing as part of Step 12. You are not the only one, however, in your household that needs this information. It is often extremely helpful if your family keeps up with you as new information becomes available concerning your disease. Sometimes family members, who are not knowledgeable about the proper treatments for arthritis, will try to push you in the wrong direction. They may encourage you to do more than you should physically. This poor and counter-productive advice may even be given to you during a flare-up of your condition when you actually need to rest more. Family members usually do not have sufficient knowledge about how inflammatory arthritis behaves to advise you correctly. If they were able to learn more by logging onto the Internet or by reading books or watching video programs, they would have a better grasp of what is truly required for you to effectively deal with your rheumatic condition. The knowledge they would receive would also make them more sympathetic as to what you are going through.

Resources on the Internet, such as those available at ArthritisCentral.com, would enable family members to understand your medications, including what side effects to expect.

Then they could assist you in monitoring your condition and help watch for any adverse reactions that you might experience.

It is often helpful to have at least one family member accompany you to the doctor's office to provide a "second pair of ears" to hear the information that the physician is providing. Sometimes the afflicted individual is so disturbed by something the doctor says that everything that follows becomes a blur. This is an excellent reason to have a second person present with you to try to glean as much as possible out of the visit. If even in spite of two people being present, you still feel that you are not able to follow all that is being explained to you at the doctor's visit, then I would suggest asking the physician if it would be acceptable for you to bring a tape recorder to your visits. That way you and your family members could review the tape recording of the visit at home and then be certain that you have understood all of the physician's explanations, interpretations of test results, and instructions. The support of your family combined with knowledge about your rheumatic condition will be an essential ingredient in your getting well and learning to take control of your arthritis.

Learning From Other Patients

Many of you will gain additional information and insights about your arthritis from fellow arthritis sufferers. This may simply come from friends who also have a rheumatic disease who call you up on the telephone to exchange information. It also may come from more formal settings. Individual support groups for the major rheumatic disorders exist in most large urban centers. This presents an opportunity for you to meet with patients with a similar medical condition to yours and to compare notes. Experts will often be invited to these meetings to make educational presentations to your group.

It is highly likely that during the course of your interactions with other patients who are sharing their experiences and knowledge that you will derive information that is pertinent to each of the 12 critical steps in taking back control of your arthritis. I would like to illustrate examples for each of these steps.

Someone that you know or meet is certainly likely to say to you, "I just found the most wonderful doctor." This may help you in Step 1 where you are trying to find a doctor you can trust. At one of these meetings or in a phone call another contact may say to you, "you know the best rheumatologist in this area is Dr. so-and-so." This will help fulfill your quest for an excellent rheumatologist in your geographic setting (Step 2). Another patient may say to you, "you know I had a great deal of pain and then Dr. X prescribed a Duragesic Patch for me, and now my pain is virtually completely controlled." Information like this can help you take back control of your pain (Step 3). Another chance interaction may have a colleague or friend state to you, "you know I couldn't take most of those NSAID medications, but my doctor put me on Vioxx and it has controlled my arthritis and does not seem to upset my stomach." Certainly, positive comments about any of the new selective COX-2 medications may influence your choice of NSAIDs (Step 4). A rheumatoid arthritis patient might say to you, "Remicade has completely changed my life and enabled me to get off of a lot of my other medications." This might prompt you to discuss this as a treatment option with your own rheumatologist. This is a component of Step 5, Take Back Control of Your DMARDs and BRMS.

A tip from a patient about switching over from methotrexate tablets to the liquid form could certainly save you many hundreds of dollars every few months. This would have impact on Step 6, Take Back Control of Your Medication Costs. You probably have many people in your family or circle of friends giving you advice on how they were able to lose weight. Weight reduction in overweight individuals is one of the numerous ways that you can accomplish Step 7, which is to Take Back Control of Your Lifestyle. A friend's recommendation about a special well-supported chair that he or she has found successful at work might persuade you to obtain a similar chair at your workplace. This is just one type of change that would be important to Take Back Control of Your Work Situation, which is Step 8. At a support group or in a telephone conversation, you are likely to have someone tell you about the most wonderful aquatics class, which is now available in your area. This would help you to Take Back Control of Your Exercise program, which is Step 9.

One of your best friends may point out to you that he or she has noted that you seem to be depressed lately. This may encourage you to discuss this diagnostic possibility with your physician and get you started on appropriate anti-depressant therapy. This is one way you may Take Back Control of Your Emotions (Step 10). Interaction with other arthritis patients in a support group may bring up issues about sexual problems affecting patients with arthritis disorders. This may prompt you to discuss these matters with your spouse when you get home. This discussion may then serve to open up communications between you and your spouse which results in improvement in your sexual relationship. Thus, by discussing this often-neglected topic with other patients, it may enable you to Take Back Control of Your Sex Life (Step 11). As more and more patients search the Internet for health sites, you can fully expect that people are going to tell you that they just discovered the most wonderful health-related website. We certainly hope that people who frequent ArthritisCentral.com feel positively enough about it to pass the word on to fellow arthritis sufferers. This will help many of you to Take Back Control of Your Information About Arthritis, which is Step 12.

It is hard, therefore, to imagine that many of you will not in some way or another be influenced by friends and family when it comes to taking back control of your arthritis and these critical twelve steps. I would like to warn you to be careful when it comes to unsupervised interactive chat rooms and discussion boards (message boards). Scams do occur on the Internet. Some individuals may not, in fact, be patients afflicted with arthritis, but individuals who are trying to sell you some unproven remedy or product. If a qualified physician is supervising a chat room interaction, then this may be helpful information for you. Be careful, however, if there does not seem to be anybody who is extremely knowledgeable or with proper credentials who is overseeing a chat room. Support groups on the other hand, usually have an affiliation with a university center, the Arthritis Foundation, or a large established rheumatology clinic in your area. Make certain that these are also run by professional individuals. Many of these will bring in qualified guest speakers who can enlighten you about your condition and this can be very educational. As with any new information that you glean from any of these contacts, the best way to find out if it has merit is to write it down or copy the resources involved and bring this information to your doctor to review it. Some lay individual may be wildly enthusiastic about some treatment, but it may not be appropriate in your case and your doctor will be able to clarify this for you.

Key Points in Taking Back Control of Your Information:

1. Acquaint yourself with a whole variety of resources available to you that deal with the rheumatic diseases, including the Internet, video programs, books, pamphlets, and lectures.

2. Become computer literate so you can take advantage of all of the information that is present on the Internet.

3. Always question and consider the reliability and veracity of information you find on the Internet.

4. Always allow your own physician to scrutinize any new information you garner from any source, and don't act on the information without your doctor's approval.

5. Use all of the resources available at the ArthritisCentral.com web site to learn the basics about the rheumatic diseases including all of the latest treatments.

6. Make sure to involve your family in this educational process so that they can assist you in taking back control of your arthritis.

7. Learn from the experiences of others who are suffering with arthritis.

8. Step by step begin the challenging task of taking back control of your arthritis. Hopefully this step-wise approach will be extremely successful for you and result in a decrease in your pain and an overall improvement in your life.

Epilogue: Now is the Time to Take Back Control

Epilogue: Now is the Time to Take Back Control

In this book, I have presented you with all of the important steps that you need to take control of your rheumatic condition. With these guidelines, you can find ways to more effectively control your pain and quiet down the inflammation in your joints. Some of you may even be so fortunate as to have your rheumatic disease go into a complete remission!

Not every step in this twelve-step approach is for every one of you. You need to consider your own situation and medical condition in order to decide whether information that I have presented applies to you or not. If you are not gainfully employed, then Step 8: Taking Back Control of the Workplace may not be a critically important step in your case. I should point out, however, that an ergonomically correct chair in your home study may still be beneficial. Also, repetitive abuse syndromes may arise from your activities in your backyard or with your household chores. Therefore, the material presented in Step 8 may still be relevant.

For those of you with osteoarthritis, Step 5 on DMARDs and biologics is not going to be helpful to you at the current time. Hopefully in the coming years there will be medications developed that will be able to truly modify or fully control your condition. If this should happen, then Step 5 will indeed become an important part of your overall strategy as well.

Everyone with a rheumatic condition certainly needs to find a physician whom he or she can trust and rely upon (Step 1). Individuals with significant rheumatic diseases should definitely find a rheumatologist who is more familiar with the newer forms of treatment (Step 2). Controlling pain and properly using anti-inflammatory medications are concerns of most people suffering with rheumatic diseases (Steps 3 and 4). Finding ways to intelligently save on the cost of medications is a universal goal

(Step 6). Patients with arthritis certainly need to evaluate lifestyle modifications that could make a big impact on their specific condition, as well as on their overall health (Step 7).

No matter which rheumatic disease you suffer from, you still need to create an exercise program that will help strengthen and condition your muscles. Every person suffering from arthritis needs to maintain the greatest range of motion possible in their joints (Step 9).

Emotional issues discussed as part of Step 10 apply to all rheumatic disease patients. Most people afflicted with arthritis will deal with issues of anxiety and/or depression at some point during the course of their illness. Marital and sexual problems also are subject matter that should be critically important to all readers (Step 11). Finally, obtaining the latest up-to-date information on new developments in your disease along with breakthroughs in treatment is your personal responsibility if you are truly going to take back control of your arthritis (Step 12).

Don't let the fear of change block your path towards taking back control of your arthritis. Step 1: Finding a Doctor You Can Trust may necessitate switching physicians. Some patients may be afraid of starting over with a new doctor. If things are not going well between you and your physician, then you need to muster the courage to make the move.

I have explained the importance of finding a knowledgeable rheumatologist if you have a significant rheumatic disease (Step 2). Instead of being more concerned with your own outcome and well being, you may be inappropriately worried that seeing a rheumatologist might somehow offend your personal physician. Most of the time, however, a good primary care doctor will actually initiate the referral to a rheumatologist when this is indicated.

Over the years I have had numerous patients who were leery of taking pain pills. They were afraid to take back control of their pain with sufficient dosages of pain-relieving medication (Step 3). Their own fears of potential addiction were interfering with their pursuit of adequate relief of their discomfort.

Some of my patients are reluctant to change their non-steroidal anti-inflammatory drug (NSAID) even though it may no longer be helping (Step 4). They are afraid of potential side-effects that might occur with a new medication. In some cases, switching to one of the newer COX-2 selective drugs may be important because of adverse reactions with traditional NSAIDs. Once again, you need to overcome your fear of change, if your physician feels you should switch medications.

DMARDs and biologics (Step 5) may be particularly "scary" to a number of you because of the potential for even more worrisome side effects. As is true in many situations with health issues, one needs to balance the benefits versus the risks involved. Don't let your fears interfere with the possibility of utilizing these revolutionary treatments to prevent joint destruction and disability, especially if your condition warrants starting on one of these newer therapies.

A fair number of patients whom I see are feeling so desperate about their situation, that they run to health food stores and spend hundreds of dollars each month on unproven remedies. They need to become more knowledgeable about these products and overcome their own fears of future disability in order to cut down on wasteful expenditures (Step 6).

Don't be afraid to make the critical modifications in your lifestyle that will help you to get better (Step 7). Make sure that you are getting adequate rest and a good night's sleep. Start to reassess your dietary intake and your need for weight reduction. Decide now that the time has come to kick the smoking habit and to cut back on your alcohol intake.

Fear of repercussions, including loss of your job, may be keeping you from speaking out at work about work-place modifications that you need (Step 8). Use all of the suggestions in this book to make your work environment more "user-friendly" to you.

If you take my advice on the "Do's" and "Don'ts" of a proper exercise program, this can be extremely helpful and you will reap the benefits (Step 9).

Don't be afraid to admit that you are feeling anxious or depressed. The vast majority of individuals suffering from arthritis are experiencing similar types of feelings. Seek out help for these problems from your doctor and don't be so reluctant to take medications that can successfully treat your emotional problems (Step 10).

Find ways to enjoy sex in spite of your arthritis. Don't be afraid to experiment with new ways of pleasuring your partner or yourself. Use the information in step 11 to bring some joy into your life and to enhance your relationship with your "significant other."

Finally, always keep searching for new information about your condition and be on the lookout for breakthroughs in treatment. Use my suggestions in step 12 (and the listings in Appendix A) to expand your knowledge. Empower yourself with this newfound knowledge.

You now have the road map laid out in front of you. Don't delay any further. Now is the time to Take Back Control of Your Arthritis. Good luck to you on this challenging journey.

Appendix A:

Internet Resources

Where to find general information about rheumatic diseases on the Internet

Website	Address	Comments
ArthritisCentral	www.ArthritisCentral.com	A comprehensive patient site with original articles and videos on the diagnosis and treatment of arthritis
ArthritisMall	www.ArthritisMall.com	A site offering educational materials including exercise and coping with arthritis
American College of Rheumatology	www.rheumatology.org	A good introduction to the most common rheumatic diseases.
The Arthritis Foundation	www.arthritis.org	A number of excellent features under "conditions and treatments"
About.com	arthritis.about.com	Has an entire section devoted to alternative or complementary medicine
AARP	www.aarp.org	Topics on fitness, disease prevention, insurance issues, and care giving.
WebMD	www.WebMD.com	Has specific sections on rheumatoid arthritis, fibromyalgia, SLE, along with other information on general health and well being.
The Mayo Clinic	www.mayoclinic.com	Check out "arthritis" under health centers listings
National Institute of Arthritis and Musculoskeletal and Skin diseases (NIAMS	www.niams.nih.gov	Under health information, click on "arthritis" or on other specific rheumatic diseases (some information also available in Spanish)
National Library of Medicine	www.nlm.nih.gov	Includes access to a great deal of information on disease states, medication, as well as other available resources.

275

Where to find specific information about rheumatic diseases on the Internet

Website	Address	Comments
The Lupus Foundation of America	www.lupus.org	This site includes research updates and educational material on cutaneous as well as systemic forms of lupus.
The Fibromyalgia Network	www.fmnetnews.com	Has educational content on fibromyalgia syndrome and chronic fatigue syndrome
The Sjogren's Syndrome Foundation	www.sjogrens.com	Has basic material about this disorder.
The Scleroderma Foundation	www.scleroderma.org	Click under "medical info" for free brochure downloads
The National Psoriasis Foundation	www.psoriasis.org	Click under "facts" or "treatment" for specific information
Spondylitis Association of America	www.spondylitis.org	Click on "about spondylitis" for further diagnostic information
The National Osteoporosis Foundation	www.nof.org	Click on "osteoporosis" or "prevention" for specific information
National Institutes of Health	www.osteo.org	Click on "fact sheets" for specific information available in English or Spanish
Drug Study Websites	www.clinicaltrials.gov www.centerwatch.com	These sites list studies being done in your geographic area that involve particular forms of arthritis.
Information on Alternative Therapies	nccam.nih.gov www.drweil.com WebMD.com altmedicine.com	These sites offer information on herbal and supplemental treatments and complementary and alternative forms of treatment

Appendix B:

Glossary of Terms

ACR 20, 50, 70—This is one of the most recent ways of measuring patient outcome in rheumatoid arthritis studies. The numbers 20, 50 and 70 refer to 20%, 50% and 70% improvement in the number of tender joints and swollen joints on exam. In addition, there are five other measurements and three out of the five also have to be improved by the same percentage. These include (1) the patient's pain assessment using a visual analogue scale of pain, (2) the patient's functional status as measured by a questionnaire, (3) an overall assessment by the patient of how they feel they are doing on a particular drug, (4) an overall physician assessment of the patient's disease activity, and finally (5) two measures of inflammation (a sedimentation rate or C-reactive protein). It is now important to be able to state at the end of a study what number of patients improved by 20% versus 50% versus 70% in utilizing these different criteria. The term ACR stands for American College of Rheumatology which is the main organization of rheumatologists in the United States and which has supported these criteria. This serves to standardize results in studies done by different investigators so that the improvement with medications can be measured by the same parameters.

Acute—Of recent onset, short lived.

Anemia—A decreased amount of hemoglobin in the red blood cells or decreased number of red blood cells which leads to a decreased ability to carry oxygen to the tissues.

Ankylosing—A joining together or fusing process across a joint.

Ankylosing Spondylitis—A form of inflammatory arthritis, which may involve the spine as well as peripheral joints. It has been associated with the gene HLA-B27.

Anti-DNA Antibodies—Very specific double stranded DNA antibodies that are found primarily in systemic lupus erythematosus and often correlate with disease flare-ups.

Anti-Malarial Drug—A type of disease modifying medication used particularly in rheumatoid arthritis and lupus. By far the most commonly used drug of this type is Plaquenil (hydroxychloroquine).

Anti-Nuclear Antibody—An antibody directed towards the nucleus of a cell (most commonly a human epithelial cell placed on a slide). These antibodies may be seen in connective tissue diseases such as systemic lupus erythematosus, but also are found in other rheumatic disorders such as rheumatoid arthritis, polymyositis and Sjogren's syndrome among others. A positive anti-nuclear antibody may even be induced by various medications or seen in association with autoimmune thyroid disease or certain liver disorders.

Arthritis—A disorder of a joint where two bones meet which may be manifested on physical examination by swelling, redness, warmth or tenderness in the joint or may be demonstrated on x-rays by loss of the joint space, formation of spurs, erosions or cysts in the bone.

Arthroplasty—A term used for the implantation of a prosthesis in a joint.

Autoimmune—Refers to the production of antibodies directed at one's own cells or tissues, a dysregulation of the immune response.

Avascular Necrosis—Refers to the loss of circulation to a portion of the bone such as in the head of the hip which leads to death of this bony tissue. This may eventually lead to a crumbling of the bone and even a subsequent loss of joint space. With avascular necrosis of the hip there frequently are x-ray changes with a flattening out of the head of the femur that is typical of this condition.

Biologic Agents—A new category of targeted therapy. Substances are synthesized which can interfere with the basic biologic and pathologic mechanisms of the disease process. These agents may interrupt the natural cascade of events, which occur in a particular disease. They may work in part by binding to various biologic messengers that are produced in disease states, or may block receptor sites where these messengers need to attach to induce further disease.

Biologic Response Modifiers (BRMs)—see biologic agents.

Bursitis—Refers to the inflammation of the bursal sacs, which are lubricating sacs adjacent to joint areas. These may simply be irritated or may actually be inflamed to the point of producing fluid within the sac with resultant enlargement. When this occurs, fluid may even need to be drained from the bursa, and corticosteroids injected in order for this to resolve.

Connective Tissue Diseases—Refers to multiple rheumatic conditions which seem to primarily affect the connective tissues of the body. These include diseases such as systemic lupus erythematosus, scleroderma (systemic sclerosis), polymyositis, or dermatomyositis.

Corticosteroids—Refers to a hormonal substance, which is found naturally in the body, but may be given by tablet or injection to help control inflammation. Currently it is the most potent of agents available to control the acute inflammatory process.

COX-1—see cyclooxgenase-1 listed below.

COX-2—see cyclooxygenase-2 listed below.

Cyclooxygenase—Refers to a particular enzyme involved in the formation of prostaglandins in the body. These may be important in the natural physiology in a particular organ or cell, or may be involved in the formation of prostaglandins that induce inflammation in a joint, in which case it may be detrimental.

Cyclooxygenase-1—(COX-1) is normally present in the body for physiologic reasons. It is also called "constitutive" cyclooxygenase. COX-1 is produced physiologically in the stomach and is protective for the lining of the stomach.

Cyclooxygenase-2—(COX-2) Refers to the "inducible" form of cyclooxygenase that arises with joint inflammation and is involved in diseases of the joints. Cyclooxygenase-2 (COX-2) is therefore produced in the joint when "induced" by inflammation.

Cytokines—Refers to biologic messenger or signaling type proteins that enable cells to influence one another. Cytokines are important as part of the immune system in the body. In disease states, however, cytokines may send messages that may lead to further joint inflammation and damage.

DMARDs (Disease Modifying Antirheumatic Drugs)—Refers to specialized medications used to control the underlying disease condition such as those used in rheumatoid arthritis.

Epidural Steroid Injection—This is an injection usually combining a form of cortisone and an anesthetic and put in the space outside of the spinal cord area. This is done to alleviate pain radiating into the leg from nerve irritation.

Erythrocyte Sedimentation Rate—A blood test to measure inflammation in the body. This is often significantly elevated in inflammatory conditions such as rheumatoid arthritis and particularly elevated in polymyalgia rheumatica or giant cell arteritis.

Fibromyalgia—A term used to describe diffuse or widespread pains involving primarily the muscles. There may be multiple tender points found on examination of these various muscle groups.

Giant Cell Arteritis—An inflammation of the blood vessels which may involve the temporal artery on the side of the head, as well as other arteries in the head area. It is often seen in association with polymyalgia rheumatica.

Gout—A condition which may be acute or chronic and which results from an excessive level of uric acid in the circulation. This results in deposits in joint areas and even in other tissues if left untreated. The release of uric acid crystals into the joint incites a significant inflammatory reaction called acute gouty arthritis.

Hyaluronic Acid—Is a substance in the synovial fluid which is responsible for the viscosity of joint fluid. It is important in the lubrication process as well as in the protection of the joint and allows for smoother motion of the joint.

IL-1—see Interleukin-1.

IL-1Ra—a natural inhibitor in the body which balances or counteracts the effects of IL-1 and is called Interleukin-1 receptor antagonist.

IL-1ra—A synthetic protein designed to counteract IL-1 (called Interleukin-1 receptor antagonist), which is currently given by daily subcutaneous injections (the small "r" denotes that it is the synthetic form of the receptor antagonist, the large "R" in IL-1Ra indicates that it is referring to the naturally found receptor antagonist in the body).

Inflammation—A process in the body tissues where all of the bodies' immune defenses including white blood cells and macrophages are drawn into one or more areas in response to tissue injury. The result of this activity may eventually lead to repair and resolution of the disease process or may even contribute to further tissue injury if not eventually treated and controlled. It is important to note that inflammation is not the same as infection and in fact in the majority of situations inflammation occurs in the absence of any live microorganisms.

Infusion—A technique of administering fluids after inserting an intravenous line in the patient's vein.

Interleukin-1 (IL-1)—A protein (also called a cytokine) that facilitates communication between cells.

Lumbar Spine—The equivalent of the low back which starts where the thoracic spine ends and goes down to the tailbone area. There are usually five lumbar vertebrae (L1 thru L5).

Myalgias—Muscle aching.

Neuropathy—Disease of the peripheral nerves. This is a common complication of long-standing diabetes mellitus, but may also be seen in association with rheumatic conditions such as rheumatoid arthritis or forms of vasculitis.

Nodule—A small node or knob-like area of tissue; in rheumatoid arthritis patients may develop rheumatoid nodules, especially over the forearms, which are often associated with a more aggressive form of arthritis.

NSAIDs (Nonsteroidal Anti-Inflammatory Drugs)—Medications used to control inflammation in the various forms of arthritis.

Osteoporosis—Disease of the bone which may lead to increased risk of fracture and is characterized by a decreased density of the bone as measured by a bone densitometer (DEXA). It involves the bone itself and is not a form of arthritis.

Patella—Kneecap.

Pleurisy—Inflammation of the lining of the lung cavity (pleura). This may occur in some patients with SLE. Also involvement of the pleura with pleural fluid production may occur in rheumatoid arthritis.

Polyarthritis—Refers to inflammation in multiple joints.

Polymyalgia Rheumatica—Is a disease primarily seen in patients over age 65 which involves pain in the muscles of the upper arms and thighs with generally a very high sedimentation rate. Some patients with polymyalgia rheumatica also may develop a more significant condition called giant cell arteritis (temporal arteritis).

Polymyositis—An inflammatory disease of the muscles associated with significant weakness.

Pseudogout—An acute inflammation of the joint induced by calcium pyrophosphate crystals.

Psoriatic—Relates to psoriasis, a skin condition characterized by scaling type skin lesions seen over the scalp, elbows, knees, and trunk; associated with arthritis in approximately 10 to 15% of cases.

Raynaud's Phenomenon—A significant color change in the digits of the hands or feet generally brought on by cold temperature or emotional upset with whitish or purplish color changes in the digits. This may be seen on its own or in association with other rheumatic conditions such as scleroderma or systemic lupus erythematosus.

Reiter's Syndrome—A condition usually consisting of three components including inflammation of the urethra, pus and inflammation in the conjunctival portion of the eye, and acute arthritis mainly in the lower extremities.

Renal—Refers to the kidney.

Rheumatologist—A physician who specializes in the diagnosis and medical management of all forms of arthritis and other musculoskeletal disease including the diagnosis and treatment of osteoporosis, chronic forms of neck and back pain, bursitis and tendinitis. A stricter definition is a physician who has completed training in internal medicine and then completes a two year fellowship in the specialty area of rheumatology. After completion of the two years of training, the physician is considered board eligible. If the physician then passes a specialty board examination in rheumatology, he or she is then considered board certified in rheumatology.

Sciatica—Pain radiating down a leg usually due to nerve irritation in the lower back area. Sometimes electrical sensations are associated with it.

Subcutaneous—Refers to the tissues just under the surface of the skin.

Synovium—Refers to the lining of the joint.

Synovitis—Inflammation of the synovial lining tissue as is seen in inflammatory arthritis such as rheumatoid arthritis.

Temporal Arteritis (also known as Giant Cell Arteritis)— Inflammation of the blood vessels over the temporal portion of the scalp (on the side of the head) which may be seen in association with polymyalgia rheumatica.

TNF—see tumor necrosis factor.

Trigger Finger—A snapping, triggering, or locking of a finger, which occurs with inflammation of tendons involved in bending or flexing the finger.

Tumor Necrosis Factor (TNF)—A protein (also called a cytokine) which is involved in biologic functions in the body and which helps in cell-to-cell communications or messaging. It is one of two principal cytokines (the other being IL-1) involved in heightening the inflammation and subsequent structural damage seen in inflammatory forms of arthritis.

Vasculitis—Inflammation of the wall of the blood vessels in the body which may then lead to changes in the flow of blood to various organs with resultant tissue damage.

Viscosupplementation—A procedure currently approved for use in osteoarthritis where viscous fluid is injected into a joint (currently the knee joint), which results in decreased pain and increased mobility. Currently available products are Synvisc, Hyalgan, and Supartz.